MW01235034

The Dash Diet

Restore Your Blood Pressure Through Weight Loss: You Can Say Goodbye To Your Hypertension By Eating Your Favorite Food Every Day

Alexander Phenix

TABLE OF CONTENTS

INTRODUCTION 6

CHAPTER 1: WHAT IS THE DASH DIET AND HOW DOES IT WORK? 9

How Dash Diet Works...14

DASH Diet And Loss Of Weight 15

CHAPTER 2: WHAT ARE THE BENEFITS OF THE DASH DIET?...17

CHAPTER 3: DOES IT WORK FOR EVERYONE?....................... 22

CHAPTER 4: IS ANYTHING WRONG WITH THE DASH DIET?.. 27

The Effects Of Being On A Dash Diet 32

CHAPTER 5: WHAT FOODS LOWER BLOOD PRESSURE AND MAKE UP THE DASH DIET?.................................... 37

Benefits of the DASH Diet: 42

CHAPTER 6: DASH DIET EATING PLAN 48

CHAPTER 7: DASH DIET RECIPES 53

1. Roasted Apples... 55

2. Banana Pancakes... 56

3. Vanilla French Toast 57

4. Raspberry Yoghurt 58

5. Homemade Sweet Corn Relish 59

6. Braised Artichokes 60

7. Simple Lentil Sauté... 61

8. Italian Style Baked Zucchini Chips.................. 63

9. Black Bean Soup 64

10. Carrot Soup... 66

11. Chicken Oatmeal Soup 67

12. Pork Soup 68

13. Red Quinoa Edamame 70

14. Grilled Salmon Cheese Salad 71

15. Fattoush Salad 73

16. Mediterranean Couscous Salad 75

17. Chicken Piccata.. 77

18. Herb Crusted Turkey Tenderloin 78

19. Oven-Roasted Turkey 79

20. Tenderized Vinegar Chicken 81

21. Herb Roasted Chicken Breast..83

22. Sole With Herbed Butter 85

23. Lemon Rosemary Salmon 86

24. Tuna Melt Zucchini Boats 87

25. Baked Cod 89

26. Mushroom Florentine Pasta...90

27. Sweet Potato Balls.. 91

28. Shepherd's Pie..92

29. Double Choc Vanilla Brownies......................................94

30. Grilled Peaches 95

CHAPTER 8: FREQUENTLY ASKED QUESTIONS 96

CONCLUSION 104

Welcome dear reader I have good news for you!

If you like reading new books in eBook format, in paperback and listening to audiobooks on the go, I have great news for you. You can sign up for **FREE**to **Alexander Phenix's** private Facebook group!

You are free to leave an honest review of your book on the Amazon platform once the reading is complete.

See below for more details!

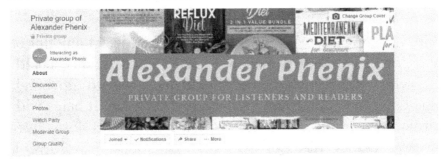

What are the benefits of the private Facebook group?

- A community of readers in which you have the same interest
- Opportunity to periodically receive new books in eBook format, totally free
- Periodically receive exclusive codes in audio format to get your audio book totally free
- All the advances on upcoming releases of new books and audiobooks
- Totally free periodic content related to a good lifestyle
- And much more

Click the links below to get started!

Alexander Phenix Facebook page

Private group of Alexander Phenix

INTRODUCTION

Which one would you prefer: to control your high blood pressure, receive costly medications with harmful side effects for the rest of your life, or turn to a proven diet, which will help normalize your blood pressure in around two weeks?

It sounds dumb, but millions of people continue to receive blood pressure drugs when they can improve their condition by adopting the DASH diet as part of their care.

With its emphasis on various foods and the correct amount of nutrients, the DASH diet can help with various health problems. DASH reflects nutritional measures to stop high blood pressure, but it may contribute even more. It helps with cardiovascular disease, strokes, diabetes, weight loss, liver disease, kidney disease, and showing you how to live a healthier lifestyle.

This diet has been applauded so much because it provides recommendations that physicians already prescribe. Guidelines such as those concerning the intake of less treated beef, sugar, saturated fats, refined fat, trans fat, and cholesterol.

Recent dietary studies funded by the National Heart, Lung, and Blood Institute have been carried out. One research investigated the impact on blood pressure from consuming a diverse, balanced diet like DASH versus eating a traditional American diet. Results have shown that healthy food, fruits and vegetables, and low-fat dairy can decrease blood pressure following a DASH diet.

DASH diet also lets you minimize fried foods, candy, and red meat. It should be noted that participants in this study decreased blood pressure even without salt intake limits. In another study, sodium limits were imposed. These participants further reduced their blood pressure.

The DASH diet works in many ways to reduce blood pressure. Firstly, high salt, highly refined foods are substituted by good alternatives, such as fruits and vegetables. Sodium-free diets are associated with elevated blood pressure, leading to heart disease, liver disease, kidney disease, and stroke. Many reports recommend maintaining your sodium intake at or below 1.500 mg per day. This is around 2/3 tea cubic meters of salt by using salt-free seasonings and by searching for and using a salt replacement.

The DASH diet is also high in nutrients, including fiber, calcium, potassium, and magnesium, with hypertension-related deficits. Ninety-eight percent of all Americans have potassium shortages. Potassium sources include beans, legumes, nuts, milk products, fruit, and vegetables.

The diet recommends daily servings of 7-8 grains, 4-5 portions of fruit and vegetables, 2-3 portions of low-fat milk and no more than two portions of meat, and 4-5 portions of beans, seeds, and nuts per week.

These recommended portions can easily be achieved by making a few simple adjustments to your diet. By adding them to salads or soups and chopping or dice as snacks, you will increase the veggie-to-meat ratio in your diet. You can choose bread, rice, and pasta versions of whole grain.

For your cereal or salad, consume nuts in your yogurt or salads with snacks of dried fruit and nuts. Replace low-fat milk with coffee and smoothies. For breakfasts, sandwiches, or salads and vegetables, use low-fat yogurt and cheese.

The DASH diet is a balanced, high-fiber diet that leads to lower blood pressure and high cholesterol. It's a balanced weight loss diet, and it's good for you when you choose a healthy lifestyle.

This GUIDE provides recipes and offers advice on how calorie intakes should be changed for weight loss. It also provides valuable tips to reduce your blood pressure by improving your lifestyle positively.

Let's get started

CHAPTER 1:
WHAT IS THE DASH DIET AND HOW DOES IT WORK?

Dietary Approach to Stop Hypertension or DASH strategies is a diet for people who want to avoid or treat high blood pressure and reduce their risk of cardiovascular disease.

The DASH diet concentrates on fruit, whole grains, vegetables, and meats. The diet was created after researchers found that high blood pressure was much less common in people who consume a herbal diet, including vegans and vegetarians.

The DASH diet emphasizes vegetables and fruits with some lean protein sources such as fish, chicken, and beans. Scientists believe that one of the most significant explanations for this diet is that it reduces salt consumption.

This diet, also known as the 'healthy diet,' is intended to offer a real solution to high blood pressure by recommending a diet that simply controls the consumption of nutrients and does not change the common diet we're used to.

Dietary methods to avoid hypertension or Dash control the sodium and fat intake to maintain an individual's natural blood pressure. Dash aims to prepare a diet that serves nutritious meals, thus stopping people from eating between meals and causing food intake loss of control. As it prevents people from starving between meals, it hopefully becomes more satisfying and less controlled.

The Dash diet teaches people to complete a specific diet program by loading the kitchen with recommended food, preparing certain meals and completing some workouts. Meal plans suggested by Dash typically contain high fiber, calcium, magnesium, and potassium ingredients. Dash diets go low on sugar and sodium and stress the need to consume green leafy fruits and vegetables.

Avocado dip is one of today's most popular Dash diets due to its very convenient and inexpensive preparation. Among the many fruits highly recommended for the Dash diet, avocados are a very rich source of monosaturated fat and lutein (antioxidants that help protect vision). Avocado should be mashed and used in this recipe, mixed with fat-free sour cream, onion, and hot sauce. This dip is eaten with tortilla chips or vegetable slices.

A total of 65 calories, 2 grams protein, 5 grams of fat, 4 grams of carbohydrate, 172 milligrams of potassium, and 31 milligrams of calcium may be derived from this dish. We may deduce that a person is fed a significant amount of required nutrients, vital to maintaining a healthy, heart-friendly diet.

Dash's dietary followers will experience normal blood pressure in just 14 days, with fewer tendencies to eat intermediate meals, which is the main culprit for weight gain. The Dash Diet Program also enables people to assess the correct amount of food consumption and exercise required, according to age and activity level.

Dash educates and inspires one of the most important reasons it is easy for people to adhere to their diet. Furthermore, the diet does not require us to give up something necessary for our daily diet, but it helps us build by adapting to little changes to support ourselves effectively.

The Dash diet is believed to prevent cardiovascular diseases, diabetes, and colon cancer. With its goal of instilling the lesson of salt in the common person's mind quickly, it has been able to help save more than 40 percent of people with hypertension lives.

Our foods affect our overall health. A diet rich in unhealthy factors such as saturated fats and cholesterol is a healthy way to treat high blood pressure and other diseases. A proper food option will decrease the risk of contracting these diseases.

The DASH diet is a clear diet that has been shown to reduce hypertension or elevated blood pressure. The diet is referred to as the DASH or nutritional strategy to avoid high blood pressure. The DASH diet is the product of research performed by researchers of the National Institute of Heart, Lung, and Blood (NHLBI). Researchers found that diets that are high in potassium, magnesium, calcium, protein, and fiber and low in fat and cholesterol can reduce high blood pressure significantly.

Three essential nutrients are also stressed in the DASH diet: magnesium, calcium, and potassium. These minerals are intended to minimize high blood pressure. A standard 2,000-calorie diet includes 500 mg magnesium, 4.7 g potassium, and 1.2 g calcium. It is very easy to adopt the DASH diet and takes little time to pick and prepare meals. Foods high in cholesterol and fats are avoided. Dieters should eat, as much as possible, vegetables, fruit, and cereals.

Provided that the foods consumed in a DASH diet are high in fiber content, you can slowly raise your fiber-rich food intake to prevent diarrhea and other digestive problems. By consuming an additional portion of fruit and vegetables in each meal, you will gradually increase fiber consumption.

Grains and B-complex vitamins and minerals are also healthy sources of fiber. Whole grain, pieces of bread, whole wheat bran, wheat germ, and low-fat breakfast cereals are some of the cereals you should eat to improve your fiber.

The food you consume can be picked by looking at the product labels of processed and packaged foods. Find low-fat, saturated fat, sodium, and cholesterol foods. The key sources of fat and cholesterol are meats, chocolates, chips, and fast foods, so you must reduce these foods' intake.

If you wish to eat meat, limit your meal to just six ounces a day, close in size to a card deck. In your meat dishes, you can eat more fruits, cereals, pasta, and beans. Low-fat milk or skim milk is a significant protein source without excess fat and cholesterol.

For snacks, you should try both fresh and canned fruit. Safe snacks are also available for people on the DASH diet, such as unsalted nuts, graham crackers, and low-fat yogurt.

Among many health benefits, the DASH diet is popular because special foods and recipes are required. The DASH diet is a balanced eating plan that focuses more on the three main minerals expected to improve blood pressure concerns.

The DASH diet is perfect for people who want warmth and ease of food. The DASH diet provides a tried and tested nutritional framework of empirical evidence for those seeking good health.

You should consider using the DASH diet if you are already suffering from high blood pressure or hypertension. You will need to talk to your doctor before deciding if you want to start a DASH diet to ensure it is right for you. Your doctor may also help you make the right decisions to ensure that your DASH diet succeeds.

As previously stated, you should eat foods high in calcium, magnesium, and potassium to be effective in your diet. Examples of foods rich in these three nutrients are fruits, vegetables, nuts, and milk products with low-fat content. However, taking supplements instead of eating these foods won't help you reduce your high blood pressure. These nutrients must be consumed from natural foods.

You will probably want to increase your intake of whole-grain foods and reduce the amount of sodium in your diet, in addition to eating a lot of fruits and vegetables. Fish and poultry can also be included in your diet but it is best to consult your doctor to find out what is the right amount for you.

It can be a bit of a challenge, like beginning any other diet, but you will excel if you take baby steps rather than make a huge drastic shift. Many times, if you do all at once, you tend to miss the foods you enjoyed but couldn't have anymore, and you give up. You can make your diet a part of your everyday routine by doing it slowly.

The way to take baby steps is to include some of your regular meal diets and set your own goals. For example, you can purchase ready-made crust, add low-fat cheese, and add loads of nutrients such as broccoli, tomatoes, and spinach to your pizza. Or, instead of oily potato chips, you could have raw vegetables with lower-fat yogurt dip. As for setting targets, you can tell yourself that you plan to snack at least one fruit each day rather than cookies or sweets.

If you have high blood pressure, the DASH diet is probably worth doing. Be sure that you consult the doctor to see how you can do that and follow the doctor's instructions. Healthy eating and a good fitness schedule will help you minimize your high blood pressure.

How Dash Diet Works

This is the nutritional strategy to avoid and even treat high blood pressure. This diet has existed for the past ten years now, and it works most of the time, according to a variety of accounts. In reality, a study shows you the results you are looking for after eight weeks of following this diet. The diet is tailored if you adopt it to reduce high blood pressure. The diet demands that you remain free from foodstuffs high in sodium.

This means you can skip the processed foods you usually purchase for your family. Various rules should also be followed if you incorporate DASH to control high blood pressure into your lifestyle. The diet also includes a reduction in total fat and saturated fat intake. If any of the foods that contain these cannot be avoided, you must restrict your fat intake.

Veggies and fruits are also popular in this diet and this high blood pressure management tool. The diet advises you that selected fruits and vegetables must be included in your diet. It is also recommended to get at least eight to ten portions of salads and vegetables high in potassium. Bananas are a great source of potassium, and this can be used in your diet.

It is also a rule in DASH that you are only serving low-fat dairy products correctly. Something excessive is also harmful to your body. Low-fat products are high in magnesium and calcium and eating three portions of these foods will help your body get the required dietary supplies of magnesium and calcium every day. For more specific food guidelines, see below some of the food products you need to consider to control high blood pressure. The foods to include in your diet are:

• Beans, nuts, and poultry in their entirety.

Consume legumes and beans, too.

• Stay away from processed food products such as frozen foods, tuna and corned beef and say no to junk and snack food.

• As stated, fruit and vegetables rich in potassium must be included. The fruit guideline is up to ten portions of fruit and veggies, and only three portions of low-fat dairy items should be included.

With these, it's easier for you to ensure that you have a balanced lifestyle and fun when you decide to control high blood pressure. The DASH diet is what you need as it advises you on the foods that minimize blood pressure.

DASH Diet And Loss Of Weight

With increased physical activity, you will lose weight when adopting the DASH diet plan at lower calorie amounts. The easiest way to lose weight is to gradually get more physical exercise and consume a healthy diet lower in calories and fat.

Physical exercise can be carried out for 30 minutes at the same time or for 3 different intervals of 10 minutes each. Try taking about 60 mins a day overall to prevent weight gain.

To encourage weight loss, the DASH Eating Plan can be implemented. It is abundant in foods with lower calories, such as fruit and vegetables. You will reduce the number of calories by swapping higher calorie foods like candy for more fruits and vegetables and making it easier for you to meet your DASH goals. Such instances are as follows:

1- Instead of four shortbread cookies, eat a medium apple. You're going to save 80 calories. Eat a fifth of a cup of dried apricots rather than a twin bag of pork rinds. You're going to save 230 calories.

2- Have a hamburger, 3 oz of meat rather than 6 oz. Put a 1/2 cup of carrots and a 1/2 cup of spinach. You're going to save over 200 calories. Stir in 2 oz of chicken and 11/2 cups of raw vegetables instead of 5 oz. of chicken, using a little vegetable oil. You're going to save 50 calories.

3- Increasing fat-free or low-fat milk products: have 1/2 cup serving of frozen low-fat yogurt rather than 1/2 cup serving full fat ice cream. You're going to save about 70 calories.

4- Other tips to save calories:

Use fat-free condiments. Use half as much soft margarine vegetable oil, or liquid margarine, or salad dressing or mayonnaise, or select low-fat or fat-free options available. Eat smaller servings and eventually cut back.

Choose milk and dairy products: fat-free or low-fat. To compare the food labels of processed goods and products with free of fat or reduced fat content, they are not necessarily lower in calories than normal versions. Limit foods with plenty of added sugar, such as pies, flavored yogurts, chocolate, ice cream, sherbet, daily fruit, and soft drinks.

Add fruit to plain low-fat or fat-free yogurt—fruit snacks, sticks of vegetables, popcorn, or rice cakes unbuttered and unsalted. Drink water or soda and zest with a lemon or lime slice.

CHAPTER 2:
WHAT ARE THE BENEFITS OF THE DASH DIET?

The DASH diet or hypertension stop strategy is prescribed, researched, and used by a doctor to reduce blood pressure in two weeks. Today, one in four Americans (about 73 million) have high blood pressure.

Blood pressure is the pressure between the artery walls, and hypertension can be characterized as a persistent rise in blood pressure. High blood pressure makes it tougher for the heart and is the principal cause of heart attack and stroke. Reduced sodium intake and balanced eating will help minimize the risk of hypertension. That's what the DASH diet is all about.

Two trials of this diet have been performed by the National Heart, Lung, and Blood Institute. These results have revealed decreased blood pressure with a diet low in saturated fat, low cholesterol, high in total fat, and high in fruits and vegetables, products free of fat or milk, whole grain, fish, and poultry.

As you can see, this diet makes more food items than most commercial diets available. They also suggest that lean red meat, candy, added sugar, and sugar-containing drinks are reduced, not removed.

Foodies would not have trouble adapting to this diet, as common food in the American pantry is not eliminated. Recipes and food plans are proposed in the DASH Diet Plan for a sodium intake of 2,300 mg and 1,500 mg.

The National High Blood Pressure Education Initiative and the United States Dietary Guidelines suggest around 2.300 mg of sodium. Compared to other food strategies for the short-term, the DASH diet also provides advice about concentrating on the diet.

Think long-term.

While weight loss is not a priority, it is a welcome impact since the DASH diet is based on a daily limit of 2000 calories. Such tips for reducing sodium more in your diet include:

Read labels of food. The amount of sodium to be contained in low-fat or refined foods can surprise you.

Please, no extra salt. When boiling pasta or rice, it is common that we add a "dash" of salt.

Find other herbs or spices in your regular recipes to replace salt.

A tea cubicle contains 2.300 mg of sodium as a tip.

It is also better to gradually make this transition because certain detoxifying reactions, such as the lack of an appetite, will stop you from doing so. It is also good to add some physical training and to have adequate medical supervision. The DASH diet provides plenty of space for longer, healthier life benefits.

Many diabetes diets have been developed to help people with diabetes control it better. However, how effective are these diets, exactly?

As the list continues to grow longer over the years, it also leaves a frustrated public wondering where to start. So I wanted to review the most popular diets on the market today, and at the end of this review, two diets were seen as excellent performers to help people control their diabetes.

One of them is the DASH diet. What's next is a snapshot of what I've heard about dieting. But you might wonder before we go into it, what exactly is a healthy diabetic diet?

It is low in carbohydrates or provides a way to balance the carbohydrate throughout the day or "burning" the excess via exercise.

It should be rich in nutritional fiber, which has proven to have many health benefits, such as a low glycemic index and a lower risk of heart diseases.

It should be low in salt. Salt can lead to high blood pressure, so reducing it is a must.

It should be low in fat. As foods easily converted to fat as sugars can make the person overweight, a risk factor for diabetes, the low-fat content of such foods is also important.

A healthy diabetic diet should aim to fulfill the recommended daily potassium allowance. Potassium is important because it can help reverse the harmful effects of salt on the circulatory system.

The DASH diet has all these features and more. But what is the DASH diet, and how did it start? In 1992, the DASH diet was formulated. Under the United States' aegis, The National Health Institute, with five of the most regarded health research centers in the United States, has collaborated to explore the impact of diet on blood pressure. This study culminated in the creation of the DASH diet, the perfect diet for balanced blood pressure.

But that's not so far from its advantages. The DASH diet was also found to be the best one for diabetes. Currently, in a study of 35 diets carried out by U.S. News and World earlier this year, the Biggest Loser diet was the best diet for diabetes. In line with many of the American Diabetes Association's advice, diabetes prevention and control qualities have been shown.

Prevention has shown that it encourages people to lose weight and hold them away. Since excess body weight is a major risk factor in developing type 2 diabetes, this consistency shows that it is a perfect alternative to diet for diabetes.

Besides, the risk factors associated with metabolic syndrome are often decreased by combining the Dash diet and the calorie restriction, which raises the likelihood of developing diabetes.

As for regulation, the findings of a small study published in a 2011 edition of Diabetes Care showed that DASHtype 2 diabetics lowered their A1C and fasting sugar levels after eight weeks. Besides, the diet is more flexible than most, making it easier to follow and adapt, following the diabetic patient's dietary advice.

Another value of this diet is its compliance with dietary guidelines. Light as it appears, it is very necessary since certain diets limit certain foods, thus leaving the person with certain nutrients and minerals potentially deficient.

This compliance breakdown reveals that the fat intake is satisfactorily reduced by 20 to 35 percent of the government's prescribed daily calories. It also reaches the 10% maximum saturated fat threshold by dipping well below that threshold. The prescribed quantity of proteins and carbohydrates is also reached.

As far as salt is concerned, this mineral has guideline meal caps. The recommended daily maximum of 2,300 mg is 1500 mg, whether you are African-American, 51 years of age or older, or under high blood pressure, diabetes, or chronic kidney disease.

This diet also properly takes care of other nutrients. This diet provides well for the recommended daily intake of 22 to 34 grams of fiber in adults.

Also, potassium is a nutrient distinguished by its ability to fight salts that improve blood pressure, reduces the risk of developing kidney stones, and reduces bone loss impressively because of the difficulty in having a recommended daily intake of 4,700 mg or 11 bananas per day.

The minimum daily intake of vitamin D is penciled at 15 mg for adults who don't get enough sunlight. Also, it is suggested that this can easily be accomplished by having cereal fortified with vitamin D.

Calcium is also good for strong bones and teeth, blood vessel development, and muscle function. The government guideline of 1,000 mg to 1300 mg is easily met here. The same applies to the B-12 vitamins. The recommendation of the government is 2.4 mg, and the supply of diets is 6.7.

While it is the second biggest loser diet to do so, it has the advantage that it was specifically formulated to help lower blood pressure and is equally effective. Therefore the DASH diet is highly recommended if you're looking for a great diabetes diet.

CHAPTER 3:
DOES IT WORK FOR EVERYONE?

The DASH diet has been designed to help people minimize or control their blood pressure without pharmaceuticals. This type of eating has also been shown to minimize blood cholesterol levels, lower inflammation, and increase insulin sensitivity. Over time, these dietary changes will help reduce the risk of stroke or heart disease.

DASH stands for Dietary Approaches To Stop Hypertension. The food plan focuses on healthy foods such as vegetables, greens, low-fat milk products, nuts, seeds, legumes, and less meat, poultry, and fish. DASH is effective as it provides good quantities of essential nutrients - nutrients that influence blood pressure - such as potassium, calcium, and magnesium.

Remember that you should change your lifestyle to reduce your blood pressure and boost your heart health. Some improvements include not smoking, low consumption of alcohol, and daily exercise.

The foods recommended for the DASH eating plan are, of course, low in sodium because it can decrease blood pressure so effectively. The article research described above is one of many proofs of the advantages of this way of eating.

Many people who want lower blood pressure search for a solution to their lifestyle, and with good reason. Experts agree that safe lifestyle changes will overcome up to 95 percent of high blood pressure issues, and diet is perhaps the most critical among lifestyle issues. In reality, diet is so important to blood pressure that it has a whole nutritional strategy: the DASH diet.

The cleverly called DASH plan is the contemporary balanced diet that we have all come to know and love: low-fat and high fiber, with a particular focus on minimal salt or sodium. But is DASH the ideal solution to blood pressure reduction? Let's look at some dietary aspects.

The first and most striking aspect of your study is that you limit all-fat (i.e., natural) milk products while studying diet for lower blood pressure. This advice is so universal and strident that any claim against it is difficult to imagine. All milk foods must also be lethal!

The low-fat diet theory has been so firmly known that it has become the backbone of modern nutrition. But from the dairy boards, you will not learn this; after all, low fat or non-fat goods are much more profitable.

Modern milk has become an abomination. Pastoral depictions of smiling cows who chew new green grass are total fiction. Cows spend most of their lives in modern mega-farms confined in large granaries with concrete floors. When they live, the vast majority of male calves are killed at birth due to their lack of milk.

Besides, ethical issues could warn you about the milk and its derivatives shipped to your local grocery store. I might go on with the growth hormones and antibiotics pumped into these unlucky cows, but let's focus on when the milk leaves the cow.

For most people, pasteurization is a method that destroys bacteria in near-boiling milk. Many people do not know that pasteurization often kills almost every other material in milk, or else it ruins it. These include the "good bacteria that support the gut and help us to digest milk first. Heating killed nutrients often provide a significant number of essential vitamins, amino acids, and minerals.

After pasteurization, milk's low nutritional value is further reduced by homogenization and the processing needed to turn milk into a low or non-fat food. To add to the injury, milk manufacturers are now attempting to restore milk to some half-food by replacing nutrients that have been lost by processing. These substitutes are marketed with pseudo-health statements such as "calcium-fortified" and "enriched with Vitamin-D."But what does blood pressure have to do with this?

Blood pressure is vulnerable to blood chemistry changes. Stable blood chemistry depends on a healthy nutrient balance, especially minerals that are processed from milk.

But is milk not "fortified" today with vitamins and minerals?

Yeah, but many scientists argue that the body does not consume nutrients from all-natural foods in the same way that it does. In other words, a lot of supplements we take, including milk supplements, are useless!

The relationship between protein and B vitamins is another example of nutrient imbalance in milk that is low or non-fat. Also, fatty milk has a very high protein content but very poor B vitamin content. This disparity helps to accumulate homocysteine. Homocysteine is an amino acid associated with atherosclerosis, hypertension, and cardiovascular disease.

These are only two examples of the many nutritional imbalances that occur first from pasteurization and further processing. Small fat and non-fat milk and other milk items should be considered dead upon delivery. The solution to this problem applies to all forms of food: get your supply as near to the source as possible and keep it as close as possible to an entire, natural state.

An example of this ideology is raw milk, which is being promoted by many. When you cringe at the thought of raw milk, I should point out that the danger of infection is practically non-existent in modern controlled conditions, in which animals are kept in good health and inspected regularly.

Did you know that there is no lactose intolerance when raw milk is consumed?

Whole, raw milk comes with the digestive enzymes that make it easy for almost everyone to enjoy. These enzymes are killed by processing, and so many people are unable to eat our supposedly balanced milk.

The health list of raw milk benefits is as long as it is impressive. They provide steady, good blood pressure and better circulation. Naturally, raw milk is not everybody's choice and it's completely impractical for most of us simply because of a shortage of availability. However, the demand for raw milk and thus its supply would increase if given a chance.

You can forget raw milk for now, but if you want to enjoy dairy products, get it the best way: whole. Consume less if calories worry you. Your heart and blood pressure will be more content with the real thing.

You can make many tasty meals full of fiber, vitamins, minerals, proteins, and cardiovascular fats in the DASH diet with a bit of imagination. Tiny, incremental improvements will help establish a solid base for a healthier life.

If you don't know where to start, here are four tips to get started:

1. Try new recipes - the internet is a perfect place to take inspiration and try some tasty new recipes. You're sure to find many recipes you enjoy with time and experimentation.

2. Eat your fruits and vegetables - the food plants are full of color, flavor, and enjoyment. In your meals, you can find innovative ways of using fruits and vegetables. Try producing smoothies, soups, chili, veggie burgers, etc.

3. Meal planning and meal preparation – it helps to sit at the beginning of the week and find out what you want to eat.

Making this activity a routine will help you organize and save time, which is useful if you are busy! Preparing food a few days in advance or even the night before is another way to help you on this new path.

4. Get going – it is necessary to make the body healthy and will reduce blood pressure. Exercise is important. Find a physical activity that you enjoy to stay inspired. Moderate exercise for just 30 minutes a day can be helpful.

Now that knowledge is in your possession, you have the potential to transform your life in the best possible way. Switch to a pace that works for you, exercise your self-love and knowledge. Keep your mind open when trying new foods and recipes; you never know what you're going to find!

CHAPTER 4:
IS ANYTHING WRONG WITH THE DASH DIET?

The DASH diet is one of the most common healthy eating plans. It began as a research study to investigate how nutrients would impact blood pressure in foods. The study showed that a diet based on vegetables, fruit, low-fat dairy foods, and legumes could lower blood pressure. It also advocates the consumption of fish, nuts, meat, whole grains, and a small number of red meals, fats, and sweets. It is also recommended that portion control be carried out.

Another experimental research, called the Lower DASH Diet, studied how blood pressure decreases in sodium (1500 mg of sodium a day) influenced people in the Regular DASH diet and those in the traditional American diet (2300 mg of sodium a day) (3500 mg average sodium per day).

The study found that blood pressure was lowered with a decreased sodium intake for both classes of people who eat the usual American diet and those who adopt the Regular DASH diet.

Those who adopted the lower DASH sodium diet, however, reported the greatest drop in blood pressure. This study demonstrates that whatever food plan you adopt, it is necessary to reduce your salt and sodium intake.

Note: Salt reduction is one of the easiest ways to reduce blood pressure. Don't use the table salt shaker, and don't add too much salt to food while cooking. Start with salt-free seasonings and a salt substitution.

Here are some tips to proceed with this balanced diet:

If there are a few vegetables every day in your current diet, consider adding another serving at lunch and dinner.

If your nutrition does not include any fruit, add fruit to your meals or take one as a snack.

Reduce to half the salad dressing, margarine, or butter you are using now. Start with fat-free dressings of salads and other condiments.

Slowly increase your intake of milk to three portions a day. To achieve this, you might replace milk with soda, alcohol, or tea. Choose free fat or reduced-fat milk products to reduce dietary fat content.

Don't buy as much meat as in the past. If you don't have it, you won't eat it in the refrigerator. Reduce meats to two servings a day, which your body wants (approximately six ounces). A card deck is about the same size as four ounces of beef.

If your current diet contains significant quantities of meat, progressively decrease it by a third. Begin to make pasta, stir fry, pans, or recipes with less meat that focuses on beans, grains, and vegetables.

Your learning DASH diet focuses on whole grains, non-fat and low-fat milk, maize meats, vegetables, fruit, nuts, and legumes/beans. It has been developed in a therapeutic environment and is not a fad diet.

While it is simple to follow, it effectively lowers blood pressure and reduces the risk of cardiovascular disease. No other diet has the same amount of medical data endorsed. This is a basic food plan that can easily be adapted to everyone's lifestyle—starting today with small lower blood pressure and healthier heart changes.

DASH is a nutritional strategy acronym for avoiding hypertension, which simply means tips for lowering the blood pressure by foods you consume. The diet plan's idea is to direct men and women with high blood pressure to eat much healthier to reduce it and the risk of related diseases.

High blood pressure is often an issue that can potentially be avoided by achieving a healthier lifestyle, but it can only be handled once a person has it.

Blood pressure is serious and can lead to coronary artery disease, dementia, stroke, and ultimately heart failure. Imagine this, about 33% of men and women have hypertension or high blood pressure. That's one-third of the adult population, so there's a very good chance either you or someone you know will be recognized as having the problem.

The Hypertension DASH diet will help you minimize blood pressure and the risk of some of the affiliated conditions by putting down a few guidelines. One of the key requirements outlined in the weight loss plan is to reduce the sodium intake to between 2.300 and 1.500 mg per day. You can still obtain a lot of sodium, but in fact, it's not so much.

Consider some of the things that you would eat every day.

Did you know that a fourth pound of cheese contains about 1,190 milligrams of sodium?

This is effectively the whole daily allowance if you restrict yourself to 1,500 milligrams a day, and at 2,300 a day, the proposed daily portion is still over 50 percent.

If you think you will be health-conscious and you will get a salad, be warned. Condiments and dressings proved infamous for high sodium levels.

The DASH diet is not only an eating schedule, it also proposes certain safe lifestyle changes:

- Start a training plan, whether the blood pressure level is typical or not.

- Try to get physical exercise for at least thirty minutes.

- Determine your own weight loss goals.

- Do not forget to take prescription medicine for high blood pressure daily.

It is no wonder, with such logical advice, that the DASH diet is currently gaining this sort of attention. This is a smart diet that offers you the ability to lose weight and stay healthy. Those with healthy blood pressure will typically benefit from the DASH diet and adhere to the minimum sodium-eating regimen with high fiber and low fat. If you adopt this diet, you can not only shed some pounds but also save your life.

Your Blood Pressure (B.P.) is taken with the assistance of a body sphygmomanometer to determine the power your heart requires to pump blood through the bones and tissues of your body. It is divided into what is known as the systolic and diastolic pressures. The systolic pressure is the highest number, while the diastolic pressure is the lowest.

When the heart contracts, the systolic measurement is reported and should be around 120 mm Hg in a healthy adult. In contrast, the diastolic measurement is recorded when the heart relaxes and normally is around 80 mm Hg in a healthy adult. You can see this reading of blood pressure written as 120/80.

There are around three million high blood pressure adults in Australia. The biggest issue with this disorder is that you don't feel it, and it can be present with a heart attack or a stroke for many years without a diagnosis. Hypertension was historically considered a 'middle-age' disease.

The latest research indicates that high blood pressure can be reduced if we have a healthy lifestyle through a well-balanced diet that decreases excess sugar and saturated fat, increases nutrients, vitamins, minerals, and antioxidants. Following daily exercise or physical activity, the heart also helps keep the muscles healthy by making oxygen and other blood nutrients more efficient.

Some people are genetically predisposed to it, whether they have a hypertensive parent or have a heart attack or stroke in their middle ages. One or more of the following problems will raise your risk of having high blood pressure:

- Abdominal fat waste
- Strong intake of alcohol
- Strong consumption of salt
- High consumption of sugar and refined carbohydrates
- Persistent Stress
- Failure to exercise
- Sedentary jobs

The DASH diet is a dietary approach validated by quality studies. This diet contains beef, chicken, and fish with fresh fruit and vegetables (rich in omega-3 fats), low-fat milk products, nuts, and whole grains.

The diet is low in saturated fat and advises that excess sugar be removed from candy, sugar, and other fast food types. The New England Journal of Medicine published the earliest findings with the DASH diet in 1997. Since these first clinical findings have been released, many other clinical trials have reported that the DASH diet can be used to lower blood pressure.

For the following reasons, nutrition experts believe the DASH diet is effective in lowering blood pressure:

- The diet is abundant in vitamins and antioxidants.

- It is a fiber-rich diet with an abundance of low glycogenic carbohydrates.

- This kind of diet works for people who want to lose abdominal fat.

- This includes a range of raw and light-cooked vegetables, fresh fruits, low-fat milk items, meat, chicken, fish, and good nut and seeds fats daily.

The Effects Of Being On A Dash Diet

This latest trend in diets is increasingly interesting among people eager for lower blood pressure by going on the DASH diet. You will not only lower your blood pressure by following the DASH diet, you will also reduce the risk of heart disease dramatically.

Besides, the American Heart Association has recommended this diet for people who have heart attacks or high blood pressure and think of eating a healthy diet. This diet also helps you lose weight and live longer.

You will have guidelines about eating healthily in the diet and how many food portions you can eat a day. This diet's main purpose is to increase magnesium, calcium, and potassium as nutrients.

Increased vegetable intake is also important for this diet, which decreases the need for unhealthy food. This diet can lead to weight loss due to a decrease in calorie intake. This diet is also against using a lot of high sodium and processed food, which raises blood pressure and makes the diet ineffective. That is why foods such as these should be restricted and concentrated on the intake of whole-grain and high-fiber foods.

This is not meant to be a long-term option, like other diets. Follow a diet only as specified. Don't overdo it: stop when the diet plan ends or feel uncomfortable, or you don't see any results. Always consult the doctor first.

DASH involves a diet that consists of foods that have proven to lower high blood pressure or hypertension. Naturally, the DASH diet also calls for foods that contribute to high blood pressure and are well-known to be minimized.

The DASH diet is not defined by any means and is therefore widely executed. Still, the rules that DASH testing provides for people with high blood pressure have shown that they can lower their blood pressure within a matter of weeks, with drastic improvements over six months. This dramatic improvement led to the country's increasing and ongoing use of the DASH diet by doctors.

The DASH diet components are very simple and easy to follow. The vegetables, fruits, legumes, seeds, and nuts play a major role in reducing blood pressure among participants. Good cholesterol, fiber, and calories are all good elements of a healthy and well-balanced diet. Olive oil is also encouraged, and studies in the Mediterranean shows that citizens using olive oil daily have lowered blood pressure.

The low-fat foods are another healthy change to the average U.S. diet from the DASH diet. The DASH diet recommends, for example, low-fat milk and meat products such as poultry and fish. Some fish contain more fats than others so that your intake is balanced between them.

Finally, it is necessary for you every day to take many whole grain items. Oatmeal is a common option for breakfast, as are granola bars and meal snacks.

The most critical move in the DASH diet is the minimization of high blood pressure foods and products. Inactivity, too much sodium, excess weight, excess alcohol, and insufficient potassium, magnesium, and calcium are the major contributors to hypertension.

You can also note that DASH diets are also recommended for weight loss. These items are used in the DASH diet and diets for weight loss because most hypertension patients are normally overweight. Most doctors report the most common treatment for hypertension is weight loss.

The vegan diet is one of the nearest diets you can equate to the DASH diet. Many foods recommended in the DASH diet are also foods that are part of the vegan diet, explaining that hypertension is only rarely diagnosed in vegans.

Proper DASH diet data is available both from your doctor and from other online food outlets. I would certainly recommend that I study DASH diets and schedule your regular diet immediately around them. The health benefits you see with reducing blood pressure are important for better health and well-being in the short term, but they are vital in the long term.

The DASH diet helps prolong your life because your cardiovascular system cannot function under higher pressure for years than planned for it. You can also access wellness tips and detailed information on my website. My free wellness platform focuses on dietary and fitness topics to lead to a healthier lifestyle for people of all ages and types of body.

Low blood pressure is a secret assassin. If left unchecked, permanent damage may result in renal failure, heart attack, or stroke. The blood pressure is considered elevated if the higher number (systolic pressure) is higher than 140, and the base number (diastolic pressure) is higher than 90 and remains there.

However, many doctors still feel that these figures are too high. Something such as 130/80 might be what you need to reduce high blood pressure risk.

There are two forms of high blood pressure: principal and secondary. In high blood pressure secondary, something else typically triggers it, such as an overactive thyroid gland.

Most people suffer from primary hypertension, however. The cause of high blood pressure in the primary type is not possible, but the medication may still be successful, although the cause may not be established.

Basic rules for high blood pressure control

- Adjust your diet
- Keep a good weight
- Exercise
- Take prescribed medicines

There are also a few dietary strategies to start the blood pressure and help stabilize it.

Limit salt intake

Most medical experts recommend that those who are sensitive to salt should restrict salt consumption to 2,000 mg daily. Watch for hidden salt, flavored butter, seasonings, tomato sauces, condiments, and canned foods. Check with your doctor before using a salt replacement.

- Limit consumption of fatty foods.
- Try grilling instead of frying.
- Set an alcohol limit
- Over intake tends to weaken the heart muscle and induce hypertension.

- Check if the Dash diet is the best diet for you with your healthcare practitioner.

- Low-fat or fat-free milk 2-3 servings

- Meat - 4-5 Servings Daily

- Fruits - 4-5 servings

- 7-8 Portions Daily - Grain and grain products

- 2 Regular portions of meat, poultry, and fish

- Nuts, seeds, and beans - 4-5 portions a week.

- Fats and oils - 2-3 parts every day

- Sweets - 5 portions a week

CHAPTER 5:
WHAT FOODS LOWER BLOOD PRESSURE AND MAKE UP THE DASH DIET?

The DASH Diet is a weight loss strategy for moderate and responsive intake. This method becomes more common as it focuses on an approach to eating healthy in the real world.

You can eat and indulge without having to count all the calories in your diet if you follow their advice. Many restaurants support dietitians by using icons on the menus to classify fatty dishes. Diners are also given more options to choose how their food is prepared.

Research assumes that this mix of nutrients can decrease blood pressure. The DASH diet can also reduce the risk of chronic illness and maintain a healthy and safe weight.

The DASH diet encourages cholesterol and saturated low-fat foods. Cutting back on fats is needed to retain your taste of healthy food and a varied menu. Dietary methods to prevent high blood pressure or DASH have been created to help people take over their hungering habits to reduce the risks of high anxiety levels.

The fascinating fact is that it helps protect dieters against osteoporosis and common human diseases, including cancer, stroke, diabetes, and heart failure. Saving yourself from multiple risks of hypertension, use these eight foods to induce a dietary approach.

1. Foods filled with whole grains such as bread, oatmeal, cereals, pasta, and rice — the body has good energy sources.

2. Fruits and vegetables — these two meals, at least eight to 10 portions a day, are recommended for daily consumption. The rich in fiber, protein, carbohydrates, vitamins, and minerals are onions, carrots, broccoli, sweet potatoes, oranges, apples, and plums.

3. Dairy products - the three primary dairy businesses are producing the most vitamins, calcium, and protein is milk, yogurt, and cheese. During DASH reduction, fat-free or low-fat dairy products are successful.

4. Meat, poultry, and fish – meat and fish are high in proteins, vitamin-B, iron, and zinc, either refined or untreated. Prepare and cook correctly before baking, roasting or frying by taking the skin and fats.

5. Nuts, seeds, and beans—almonds, kidney beans, sunflower seeds, etc., are decent magnesium, potassium, and protein sources. They are also rich in fiber, and their phytochemicals help cure cardiovascular diseases and cancer.

6. Fats and oil-fat-enriched diets help the body consume the important immune system vitamins. Unhealthy fats can exacerbate the risk of heart disease, diabetes, and obesity.

7. Low-fat sweets—jellybeans, graham crackers, and light-flavored cookies are also considered in this consumption curriculum. Dark chocolate is also recommended because it contains fewer hypertensive substances.

8. Snacks with low sodium—buy foods with "no salt added" or "low sodium-rich" labels.

Now you want more resources, to be safer, to look younger, to lose weight, to cleanse your body, right?

Here are some key ingredients to ensure that you succeed with this very common approach;

1) Stay away from the bread, if possible – but if you're really hungry, you can have a roll without butter.

2) Ask for low fat and side dressage for salad dressing.

3) Pick the green or tossed spinach

4) Ask for your food to be prepared with olive oil instead of butter.

5) Selecting foods steamed, grilled, broiled, roasted, or stir-fried is safest.

6) Pick vegetables as side meals. Baked potatoes and rice are alright as well.

7) Skip fries and onion rings.

8) Cut off any obvious meat fat.

9) Drinking water, club soda, juice, the diet of soda, tea or coffee is best

10) Say no to excess - limit yourself to two.

13) Skip soup and choose fruit or salad instead.

14) Always be mindful of salt consumption!

15) Always stop having too much to eat!

Other items listed by the DASH diet are more visible traps that dieters fall into, like salad's paradox. Don't assume that just because it is green, it means that it's good or low calorie - some salad dressings are plain fat!

A sensible diet, yes but it will not revolutionize your figure or turn you soon into a hard body. But if you only want to be a little healthier and self-conscious, that is a small but crucial step in the right direction.

The good news for us all is that this food plan is quick to execute. It makes most food styles and requires no special or hard-to-prepare dishes.

DASH has been developed by the National Institutes of Health, based on the Mediterranean diet and study of the National Heart, Lung and Blood Institute (NHLBI) (N.I.H.). DASH, a nutritional strategy for stopping high blood pressure, is the well-researched diet in foods with lower blood pressure today.

It is about putting into our diet balanced quantities of whole-grain, meat, fish, and nuts. It makes low-fat milk products and magnetic red meats. Sweets and drinks containing sugar are reduced but not excluded.

It is abundant in potassium, magnesium, calcium and high in fruit and vegetables. Elevated fiber and protein concentrations are also included (18 percent). It is equally necessary for us to eliminate the salt shaker and find savory, healthier ways to season our food.

The diet allows you to cut down the sodium levels in your diet and indulge in food with a high potassium and calcium, and magnesium level. With strict adherence to the DASH diet, you will be able to bring down your blood pressure by a few points in just two weeks. Over time, this will go down further, taking you out of the risk list.

The DASH diet focuses on reducing your intake of sodium. The norm in this diet is an allowance of 2300 mg a day. This is much lesser than the average of 3500 mg that we appear to consume daily.

In the DASH diet, you have to include about 6 to 8 servings of grain regularly. The emphasis has to be on fiber and nutrient-based grains. Use brown rice and not white, wheat pasta, and not flour based ones.

Since grains are low in fat, keep it that way and stay away from butter and cream cheese-based sauces. Vegetables such as onions, peppers, carrots, broccoli, green are all made of fiber, vitamins and packed with healthy nutrients like potassium and magnesium.

Vegetables should be had as a main course and not as a side dish. If you are going for canned vegetables, it will be a good idea to go for a lower sodium count. Since you have to have many servings per day, it would be a good way to hone your cooking imagination.

Often, fruits ought to be part of your diet. Include fruit with your diet and even snack on it. Make sure you add a good dose of fruit to your yogurt. Include milk, particularly fatty yogurt. You should use alternatives if you are lactose intolerant.

When it comes to meat, you can stick to less than six servings a day. Your best choices are lean meat, chicken, and fish. Take the skin and fat and use cuisines such as grilling, barbecue, roasting, or poaching. You will also have to take care of your oils and reduce your alcohol intake and related items to make the most of the DASH diet.

This diet's side effect is weight loss; this is due to the healthy eating habits a person goes on to control their blood pressure.

The DASH diet aims at:

There are many different ways of food processing, and others include dehydration, canning, and freezing. There are probably many more ways to process foods, but I think you get the picture with the few examples I have provided.

Processed foods are not as safe as fresh foods; below are a few examples of the foods to avoid:

1) Canned foods [most of these canned products contain a lot of sodium]

2) White pieces of bread [made from processed wheat] are made from whole grain flour rather than consumed bread.

3) Pasta

4) Snacks like chips and cheeses.

5) Frozen suppers.

6) Frozen sticks/fresh fish.

7) Cakes and cake mix packed.

8) Cookies baked and packed.

9) Mixes of food[boxed].

10) Processed meats such as polony, Vienna, etc.

11) Some cereals for breakfast - particularly those loaded with sugar.

 Some Foods To Be Avoided:

Foods high in fat and cholesterol, like red meat, candy, and certain milk products, should be avoided to the greatest extent possible.

Benefits of the DASH Diet:

1) A decrease in substantial and diastolic blood pressure – avoiding heart disease.

2) Loss of weight - the extra advantage of the DASH diet.

3) Increased vitality – a person's balanced diet can reduce blood pressure.

Studies on this diet were performed, and the findings are available on the N.I.H. website for analysis.

According to studies released by Harvard Health Publications in 2009, 73 million Americans and 1 billion people worldwide are battling high blood pressure (the medical term for high blood pressure).

The NHLBI study found a strong correlation between cardiovascular disease, hypertension and strokes, and kidney disease. If you are between 40 and 70 years old, the risk of cardiovascular disease doubles with each 10 mm Hg in your diastolic reading or 20 mm Hg in your systolic reading.

We recognize that an unhealthy diet is one of the risk factors for high blood pressure. With one in three Americans living with hypertension, NHLBI started a study through some of the country's most recognized health facilities to figure out the best eating strategy to prevent or mitigate hypertension.

The research included a control diet that was the standard American diet and two other diets. The third diet, known as the DASH diet, was most successful. Their results: blood pressure has been lowered with a low diet plan:

- Saturated Fat
- Cholesterol
- Complete fat emphasizing fat-free milk and dairy products

There were plenty of fruits and vegetables in the food plan. In the next two weeks after the DASH eating program, doctors saw immediate improvements in blood pressure rates. We cannot overestimate these results' significance: with the DASH findings, we can now reduce the risk of two main dietary causes of heart disease and stroke - high blood pressure and cholesterol.

The second research applied to the DASH strategy a decrease in sodium (salt) consumption. Participants who followed the DASH plan and consumed 1500 mg (2/3 tsp) or less of their salt daily saw a substantial additional decrease in their high blood pressure levels.

Tips for consuming low blood pressure food

- Make your meal based on complex carbohydrates (e.g., pasta).
- Make meat a lateral dish, not the primary one.
- Eat meats, poultry, fish and lean meats.
- Eat food with a range of colors, textures, and goodies to prevent boredom and a return to old habits.
- Steam, barbecue, bake, stir-fry but don't fry.
- Eat fruit and other delicious replacements for table sugar.
- Create your seasoning mixture to produce food tastes and minimize salt.
- If you eat them, rinse off salt from canned foods and cured foods.
- Change your favorite recipes to the ideals of the DASH diet.
- Make progressive reforms.

The DASH eating plan has other advantages, such as lowering LDL (bad), reducing the risk for heart disease, and lowering blood pressure. Blood pressure is reduced alone by either approach; however, a combination of eating guidance and decreased sodium intake produces the greatest advantage that hinders high blood pressure development.

The diet plan for Dash is:

1- Poor in sugar, cholesterol, and total fat.

2 - Rich in fruits, vegetables, and milk and dairy products that are free or low in fat.

3- Full grains, fish, poultry, and nuts included.

4- Minimal in lean red meat, candy, added sugar, and drinks containing sugar relative to a traditional U.S. diet.

5- Potassium, magnesium, calcium, protein, and fiber-rich nutrients that are expected to lower blood pressure.

DASH daily nutrient targets (2100 calorie plan):

- Net fat: 27% calories
- Saturated fat: 6% calories
- Protein: 18% calories
- Carbohydrate: 55% calories
- 150 mg of cholesterol
- Soy: 2.300 mg.

The diet contains two amounts of sodium intake per day at 2,300 and 1,500 mg. The highest appropriate standard for the National High Blood Pressure Education Program is 2300 milligrams.

The less salt you ingest, the lower your blood pressure. Studies have found that the DASH menus of 2,300 mg of sodium can reduce blood pressure and that an even lower 1.500 mg of sodium can further reduce blood pressure. The current U.S. salt intake is 4,200 mg/day for adult men and 3,300 mg/day for adult women.

- Energy: 4,700 mg.
- Calcium is 1.250 mg
- Magnesium: 500 mg
- Fiber: 30 grams

The Dash Diet is advised by the U.S. National Heart, Lung, and Blood Institute and the American Heart Association. The nutritionist, Maria Heller, has created it to help lower blood pressure, minimize cholesterol, and normalize diabetes. Being on a balanced diet, everyone lost a lot of weight.

We have a successful crash diet that is approved by medical practitioners for the first time. You will then easily lose weight and improve your fitness at the same time.

No calories are counted, and no priority is put on what you can't consume. Heller is assured that you can concentrate on what you have to eat. It is a high-protein and low carb diet, with the free food being veggies. It differs from other related diets because it encourages minimal saturated fats but promotes healthy consumption of natural fats.

Your meal should include a portion of each of the following food groups.

1. Low in saturated fats, proteins.

- Little meat
- Poultry and fish
- Cheese with low fat
- Yogurt

2. For good blood circulation and cell regeneration, healthy fats are important.

Seeds and noodles

Olive oil, in particular, vegetable oils.

Rapeseed oil

3. All vegetables, except potatoes and maize.

You can eat as much as you want and all the vegetables are free.

Salads included

Phase 1 — The first two weeks will charge your metabolism by cutting most starch and sugar, including all grains and fruit. You might feel a little tired in this phase but don't be worried as it's only for a short time.

Phase 2 - Continue in the same way, but you can reintroduce some grain and fruit now that your metabolism has been optimized—a portion of whole-grain bread and a portion of fruit or fruit juice.

For the rest of your life, this phase should become hundreds of healthy recipes that support this stage, and this food plan should become your choice of life. It takes just a little organization to ensure that you always have the ingredients for your next meal; preferably, shop in advance for at least three meals. The more organized you are, the more likely you are to keep it.

CHAPTER 6:
DASH DIET EATING PLAN

DASH diet eating plan is high blood pressure non-pharmacological treatments. It is part of lifestyle changes, including low intake of saturated fat, increase intake of vegetables and fruit, additional carbohydrate-containing products such as whole-grain products, increased food intake for fish, poultry, and nuts.

A study has shown that the DASH diet plan has the most impact on blood pressure and cholesterol reduction than a normal diet. The result can be seen two weeks from now!

Tips For DASH food ingestion with lower calories Plan!

1. Fruit increase

An apple keeps the doctor away for one day! In the dietary plan, apple and dried apricots are the best choices for high blood pressure patients.

2. Vegetable Increase

Hamburger! Yes, even if it is a favorite food for most people, it could increase your blood pressure. It's very difficult for you, I know, to stop eating it. However, I would suggest that you weigh 3 ounces of meat rather than 6 ounces of larger size.

This is also when chicken consumption with only 2 ounces of weight is reduced and accompanied by a raw vegetable plate.

3. Increase milk products free of fat or low-fat

For instance, traditional ice cream can be replaced with fat-free yogurt.

Salt and Sodium Elimination

With the method of ingesting more fruit and vegetables into DASH, its lower sodium content has made it easier to eat less salt and sodium. Furthermore, fruit and vegetables are rich in potassium and play a role in lowering high blood pressure. Milk products and fish are other important dietary sources.

Tips for Salt and Sodium Reduction

Restrict food high in salt. It is safest to take no or low-salt foods.

Increased vegetable consumption

No salty rice, pasta, or other mixed meals

Removal of excess salt from preserved food, such as tuna or beans, preserved in a can.

Excess body weight is closely related to elevated blood pressure. This reduces weight by lowering blood pressure in many people who have high blood pressure and are 10 percent heavier than the ideal weight.

Too much alcohol consumption can increase blood pressure and cause anti-high blood pressure therapy resistance. You should limit the daily intake to one drink for women and two drinks for men when consuming alcohol.

Regular participation in aerobics and physical activity allows both alleviating and controlling high blood pressure. Unfit individuals with normal blood pressure have a 20 percent to 50 percent higher chance of high blood pressure than their more active and fitness counterparts.

The higher your salt intake, the higher your blood pressure, and almost all Americans eat more salt. African Americans, older and middle-aged adults, and high blood pressure people are more sensitive to salt.

The DASH diet is based on two thousand calories a day. Use this guide to help you pick the food or take it to the grocery store.

* Wheat and grain products

1. Daily serving: 7 to 8

2. Serving sizes: 1 slice of bread, 1 lb. Cooked rice, pasta, cereal 1/2 cup.

3. Examples include a muffin, wheat brown pita bread, cereal, rice, oatmeal, crackers, unsalted pizzas, popcorn.

4. DASH Food Group Importance: primary sources of energy and fiber

Plants

1. Regular Servings: 4 to 5

2. 1 cup of raw leafy, 1/2 cup of vegetables, 6 oz., vegetable juice

3. Examples include tomatoes, potatoes, chocolate, green peas, squash, broccoli, gourmet turkey, frozen greens, and kale.

4. DASH Food Group Importance: rich in potassium, magnesium, and fiber source

Fruit

1. Regular Servings: 4 to 5

2. Serving size: 6 oz. 1 medium fruit, 1/4 cup of dried fruit, 1/2 cup of fresh fruit, frozen or canned.

3. Examples include: fruits of the apricots, bananas, dates, raisins, oranges, grape juice, raisin juice, mango juice, pineapples, prunes, raisins, tangerine, strawberries

4. DASH Food Group Importance: big sources of potassium, magnesium, and fiber

Fat-free dairy products

1. Serving sizes: 2 to 3 daily

2. Serving sizes: 8 oz. 1 taste of yogurt, 1 1/2 oz. milk, cheese

3. Examples include fat-free (skim) or fat-free buttermilk (1 percent), fatless or low-fat regular or frozen juice, fat-free cheese

4. DASH Food Group Importance: key sources of calcium and protein

Fish, meat, and poultry

1. Serving size daily: 2 or fewer

2. Serving size: 3 oz. Fried beef, poultry, or fish

3. Examples: pick only lean meat, eliminate visible fats, grill, bake, boil or remove the poultry skin.

4. DASH Food Group Importance: rich protein and magnesium sources

Nuts, kernels, and dry beans

1. Daily serving: 4-5 a week

2. Serving size: 1/3 cup or 1 1/2 oz. of nuts. 1⁄2 cup of dried, cooked beans, peas

3. Examples include almonds, peanuts, sunflower seeds, kidney beans, mixed nuts lens.

4. Food Group Rich energy source: magnesium, potassium, protein, and fiber

Fats and oils

1. Daily Servings: 2 to 3

2. Serving sizes: 1 teaspoon, one light dressing salad, vegetable oil, egg olive, corn, canola, or safflower

3. Examples include soft margarine, sweet mayonnaise, sweet salads, olive, corn, canola, or vegetable oil.

4. DASH has 27% fat

Sweet honey

1. Daily servings: 5 to 7

2. Servings: 1 cube of sugar, two cubes of jelly, 1/2 oz. jelly

3. Some examples include maple, sugar, jelly, jam, fruit gels, hard sweet fruit punch, sorbet, ice cream

The DASH diet recommends that 8 to 10 portions of fruit and vegetables and 2-3 portions per day of milk products should be made.

The DASH diet also contains low fat, saturated fat, cholesterol, added sugar, and limits the amount of red meat and sugar found in beverages. DASH dietary plans make it easier to consume less salt and sodium because it is high in fruits and vegetables, which are naturally lower in sodium than many other foods.

CHAPTER 7:
DASH DIET RECIPES

DASH is a diet formulated specifically to reduce blood pressure. Compared to the moderate weight-loss diets, it is not hard to adhere to and has immense advantages to control blood pressure and minimize other diseases like diabetes and cancer.

Diet plays a significant role in both developing and reducing high blood pressure. Food is the power of our body. If you think about it, a bad diet is very close to pouring gas into an unleaded vehicle.

The engine will still operate, but it will run rough and simply stop working due to carbon buildup over time. It has the same effect to fill our bodies with salt, sugar, and saturated fat.

There are two explanations for why the DASH diet plan works. First of all, it consists of foods rich in vitamins, minerals, fibers, and antioxidants, which lower pressure and reverse blood harm. Secondly, it removes junk, which caused the problem first and foremost.

Here's a short rundown of the food types you can expect from the DASH diet:

Whole grains, such as oatmeal and cereals that contain complex carbohydrates and fiber.

Fruits, such as strawberries, broccoli, beans, bananas, and berries, contain potassium, magnesium, fibrous, and antioxidants.

No fat or low-fat milk products like milk, yogurt, or cheese that contain protein, calcium, and magnesium.

Protein and magnesium, gotten from poultry, lean white meats, and fish.

Nuts and beans, including almonds and calcium, fiber, and vitamin B pistachios.

Nice fats and oils like olives, canola oil, and our fats' avocados.

You must dedicate yourself to the diet to make it work, and you can prepare it, especially for the meals you eat. However, compare this bit of work to the struggle and pain of blood pressure medications, and I believe you conclude that the effort is worth it.

In less than two weeks, you can reduce your blood pressure readings by 20 points following the DASH diet plan, combined with a bit of everyday exercise and relaxation techniques. Give it a chance; give it a try. Your heart's going to thank you.

The diet suggests how many items from each food category should be consumed every day. Calcium, magnesium, and potassium are consumed every day to improve the use of good heart minerals. When most people consume less meat and more vegetables, they reduce their calorie consumption when reducing junk food.

Naturally, reducing the daily intake of calories will cause weight loss. The diet also emphasizes reducing sodium, making it important to reduce refined foods and promote whole grains and other high-fiber foods.

Ironically, this diet is promoted by the Mayo Clinic rather than the fad three-day diet that sometimes mistakenly bears the name of the Mayo Clinic. The DASH diet is a balanced alternative to common sense food.

It is easy to obey, and you won't be left feeling hungry, although it restricts or limits certain foods. The diet is not just for people who choose to eat balanced cardiac diets. Any of the principles, such as consuming fewer processed foods, can and should be included in every diet.

1. Roasted Apples

Ingredients

1/4 cup of sugar

1/8 teaspoon of ground cinnamon

6 apples cut into quarters

Directions

Preheat the oven to 400°C. In a medium dish, mix sugar and cinnamon. Attach apples and cover—spread apples over a rimmed baking sheet in one layer. Bake, flipping, tender but strong, for 30 to 35 minutes.

2. Banana Pancakes

Ingredients

  1 cup of flour

  1 tablespoon of sugar

  2 teaspoons of baking powder

  1 egg, beaten

  ¼ teaspoon of salt

  2 tablespoons of vegetable oil

  2 mashed ripe bananas

  1 cup of milk

Directions

Mix meal with white sugar, salt, and baking powder. Mix egg, milk, vegetable oil, and bananas in a separate dish.

Add flour mixture into the banana mix.

Over medium heat, heat the lightly oiled griddle or fry pot. Pour the batter into the griddle or scoop it down, using about 1/4 of a cup for each pancake. Cook until pancakes on both sides are golden brown.

3. Vanilla French Toast

Ingredients

2 eggs

1/2 cup of milk

2 tablespoons of sugar

1 tablespoon of Pure Vanilla Extract

1/4 teaspoon of Ground Saigon Cinnamon

1 tablespoon of butter

Directions

In a medium cup, whisk eggs, milk, sugar, vanilla, and cinnamon. Melt butter over medium-high heat inside a skillet. Soak the egg mixture into bread slices and brown them in the pot on either side. Serve with maple syrup.

4. Raspberry Yoghurt

Ingredients

  2 cups of raspberries (fresh)

  1 teaspoon sugar

  2 teaspoons lemon juice

  Plain Greek yogurt

Directions

Blend raspberries, sugar, and lemon juice. Mix and mash the raspberries.

Cook at low-medium heat for around 3-4 minutes. The mixture should not be runny, and a sauce must be consistent.

Let it cool. After the mixture is fully cooled, add the desired amount to some Greek yogurt and enjoy!

5. Homemade Sweet Corn Relish

Ingredients

   10 ears of sweet yellow corn

   2 large red bell peppers,

   2 large green bell peppers

   8 ribs celery

   1 large, yellow or sweet onion

   4 cups of apple cider vinegar

   2 cups of sugar

   1 tablespoon of whole yellow mustard seeds

   3 teaspoons of salt

   4 pcs of whole allspice berries

Directions

Mix all the ingredients inside a pot and boil until the sugar is dissolved. Reduce the heat to medium and simmer until soft, while uncovered, for about 20 minutes.

Put your delicacies into hot sterilized jars and seal them with cloves. Put the jar in a water bath for 10 minutes.

Keep in a cool, dark spot. It will be held for at least one year. Store in the fridge for up to two months.

Makes about 8 pints

Note: Wait a week or two before eating to give the vinegar time to soften.

6. Braised Artichokes

Ingredients

   4 pcs of medium artichokes

   4 tablespoons of butter

   1 cup of chicken stock

   Salt

   Freshly ground pepper

   Zest and juice of 1 lemon

Directions

Break each artichoke in half; remove the hardest external leaves.

Put 3 tablespoons of butter over medium-high heat in a big, deep skillet. When it melts, add the artichokes and cook about 5 minutes until lightly browned.

Add chicken stock, cover and turn the heat to medium-low.

Cook about 20 minutes or until tender, check for enough liquid in the pan every 5 or 10 minutes, and add more stock, when necessary. Sprinkle with salt and pepper and transfer artichokes to a bowl.

Boost the heat to medium-high and cook until liquid is reduced to a sauce and stir occasionally. Stir the lemon zest and lemon juice and the remaining tablespoon of butter: taste and season. Serve artichokes with sauce.

7. Simple Lentil Sauté

Ingredients

   1 cup of lentils

   2 pcs of cloves garlic

   1-inch piece of fresh ginger

   1/2 jalapeño

   1/2 teaspoon of coriander seeds

   1/2 teaspoon of black peppercorns

   1/4 wedge of fresh lemon

   1 tablespoon of light agave

   Salt

   1 tablespoon fresh coriander

   1 teaspoon of sesame oil

   1 tablespoon of vegetable oil

   Cooked Basmati rice

Directions

1. In a mortar and a pestle, coriander seeds and black pepper grains have been broken up: ensure that you have some texture.

2. In a medium to high flame, position a medium-wide, non-stick skillet for sauce and vegetable oils. When the oil is hot, add the oils and coat in crushed spices. Add garlic, ginger, jalapeños, and more.

Pour in lentils for around 1 minute; make sure that they are strained by soaking water. Sauté for about 5-8 minutes – they start to cook and get darker in color.

3. Put in the lemon juice and agave and stir after about 8 minutes or so. Add a splash of water to steam the lentils slightly so that they cook faster. Add salt. Shake – lentils should be tender, slightly dressed, spicy, and balanced with agave sweetness.

Adjust seasonings accordingly. Take it off the heat and toss it into chopped coriander. Serve with rice.

8. Italian Style Baked Zucchini Chips

Ingredients

  1 large zucchini, sliced

  1/4 cup of olive oil

  1/8 teaspoon of garlic powder

  1/2 teaspoon of dried basil

  Kosher salt

Directions

Preheat the oven to 275°C. Line with large parchment paper cookie sheets

Into the olive oil, put the garlic powder and basil to marinate when slicing your zucchini.

Slice courgettes. Lay the courgette onto a paper towel in one layer and put another towel on top, pressing gently to extract moisture.

Brush the paper with oil gently. Place the courgettes into one layer and gently brush the tops with oil.

Sprinkle with Kosher salt gently.

Bake until the chips are crispy, or for 90 minutes.

9. Black Bean Soup

Ingredients

2 tablespoons of extra-virgin olive oil

1medium red onion

2 garlic cloves

1 tablespoon of minced jalapeños

1 tablespoon of tomato paste

Kosher salt

Freshly ground black pepper

1 teaspoon of chili powder

1/2 teaspoonof cumin

3(15-oz.) cans black beans

1 qt.low-sodium chicken

1bay leaf

Sour cream

Sliced avocado

Chopped fresh cilantro for garnish

Directions

Pour oil into a big pot over medium heat. Add some onion and cook until soft for around 5 minutes. Add jalapeños and garlic and cook for around 2 minutes. Add the tomato paste, mix and cook for about a minute longer—season to taste with salt, pepper, cumin, and chili powder.

Mix the black beans with their liquid and chicken broth. Remove the broth, add the laurel, and cook. Boil immediately and cook, about 15 minutes, until slightly reduced. Take the leaf out.

Using an immersion blender, mix the sugar to the desired consistency.

Serve with a sour cream dollop, cilantro, and avocado slices.

10. Carrot Soup

Ingredients

   1 tablespoon of butter

   1 tablespoon of extra-virgin olive oil

   1 medium onion

   1 stalk celery

   2 cloves garlic

   1 teaspoon of chopped fresh thyme

   5 cups of chopped carrots

   2 cups of water

   4 cups of low-sodium chicken broth

   ½ cup of half-and-half

   ½ teaspoon of salt

   1 Freshly ground pepper to taste

Directions

Heat butter and oil in an oven at medium heat until butter melts. Add the onion and celery, cook 4 to 6 minutes, whisking periodically until tender. Add garlic and thyme (or parsley) and cook, mix, about 10 seconds, until odorless.

Remove carrots. Add broth and water and boil over high heat. Reduce the heat and cook until very tender for 20 min.

Puree the soup in batches in a blender until it becomes smooth. Add half, salt, and pepper (use caution when pureeing warm liquids).

11. **Chicken Oatmeal Soup**

Ingredients

   1 boiled chicken breast

   1 cup of oats

   1 tablespoon of Flour

   1 small onion

   1 spring onion

   1/2 teaspoon of cumin seeds

   Salt as per taste

   1/2 teaspoon of black pepper powder

   1 teaspoon of cooking oil

Directions

In the pan, heat oil, sprinkle cumin seeds, and sprinkle onion for a minute.

Add shredded chicken and sauté for a minute.

Add salt and powder mixture in black pepper to cook for a few seconds.

Add maida and small stock of chicken (in which chicken boiled). Remove constantly and then add 1&1/2 cup of chicken stock.

Add oats and cook on low flame for 3 minutes.

Add some chicken oats spring onion soup ready to eat.

12. Pork Soup

Ingredients

  2 (8 ounces) bone-in pork chops

  1 teaspoon of paprika

  1 teaspoon of dried oregano

  1 teaspoon of garlic powder

  ½ teaspoon of salt

  ½ teaspoon of ground black pepper

  ½ teaspoon of chili powder

  1 bay leaf

  3 cups of chicken broth

  2 cups of water

  2 tablespoons of soy sauce

  ¼ cup of flour

  3 potatoes

  1 cup of chopped broccoli

  1 diced carrot

  1 diced onion

  2 diced stalks celery

Directions

In a large pot, put pork cups, oregano, paprika garlic powder, pepper, salt, chili powder, bay leaf, chicken pudding, water, and soy sauce. Boil the mixture and then reduce heat to medium-low and allow 1 hour to cool. Remove the pork chops and cool them.

Whisk 3/4 cups of the flour with the cooking liquid: set aside. Remove and discard any bones or fat if the pork chops are cool. Chop the meat into bite-size.

Add potatoes, broccoli, carrot, onion, celery, and pork to pot. Bring the mixture to a boil, and then add the flour to the blend. Reduce heat for 1 hour and cook. Join the baking leaf and mash the potatoes before serving.

13. Red Quinoa Edamame

Ingredients

1 cup of uncooked red quinoa

1 6-ounce bag of baby arugula

1 bunch of parsley

1 cup of frozen sweet peas

2 cups of frozen edamame

1 1/2 cup of canned mandarin oranges

2 cups of red cabbage

1 thinly sliced shallot

Dressing

1/2 cup of fresh lemon juice

1/2 cup of mandarin oranges

1/4 cup of virgin olive oil

1 – 2 tablespoons of honey

Salt to taste

Directions

Put 2 cups of water and quinoa in a saucepot and bring to a boil. Reduce fire, cover, and cook for 15 minutes. Fluff with a fork and set aside to cool. Drain any excess water.

Place the dressing ingredients in a blender and combine until smooth.

Dress all the ingredients in a large salad bowl, drizzle, and toss well coated.

Serve cool

14. Grilled Salmon Cheese Salad

Ingredients

 1 tablespoon of olive oil

 8 oz salmon fillet

 Salt and pepper

 4-5 spears asparagus

 2-3 cup of arugula

 2-3 button mushrooms

 1/2 sliced avocado

 1 oz crumbled blue cheese

 2-3 tablespoons toasted sliced almonds

 Pinch micro-greens

Vinaigrette

 2 teaspoons of extra virgin olive oil

 1 tablespoon of lemon juice

 1 teaspoon of mustard

 1 teaspoon of unpasteurized honey

 1 teaspoon of fresh thyme

 1/4 teaspoon of salt

 1/4 teaspoon of black pepper

Directions

Toast the sliced almonds until golden in a small pot and throw them for about 5 minutes, mostly to prevent burning. Set aside.

Heat the olive oil over medium-high heat in a non-stick pot. Meanwhile, brush salmon generously with salt and pepper on both sides. After it is hot, add the salmon fillet on one side and asparagus on the other side and cook on the fish until a pleasant golden crust is made, approximately 3-4 mins per side.

In this case, combine all dressing ingredients in a small glass container or weigh a cup of the whisk until the mixture is well and partially emulsified. Set aside.

Place in a shallow bowl or plate; top with champagne and avocado slices. When you cook your fish and asparagus, place them on top of the salad and sprinkle with sliced almonds and crumbled blue cheese. Garnish, if needed, with a pinch of microgreens.

At the moment of eating, dress the vinaigrette in your salad.

15. Fattoush Salad

Ingredients

   2 loaves of pita bread

   ½ teaspoon sumac

Olive Oil

   Pepper and salt

   1 pc of the heart of lettuce

   1 pc of cucumber

   5 pcs of tomatoes

   5 pcs of green onions

   5 pcs of radishes,

   2 cups of parsley leaves

   1 cup of mint leaves

For the Lime vinaigrette

   1 ½ lime juice

⅓ cup of olive oil

Pepper and salt

   1 teaspoon of ground sumac

   ¼ teaspoon of ground cinnamon

¼ teaspoon of ground allspice

Directions

Toast pita bread in the oven until it's crisp but not browned. In a big pot, heat 3 tablespoons of olive oil. Break the pita bread and bring it into the heated oil. Briefly fry until browned, sometimes tossing. Add salt, pepperand around ½ teaspoon.

Remove pita chips from the heat and put them on paper towels to soak the oil.

Mix cut spinach, cucumber, tomatoes, green onions with sliced radish and parsley in a large mixing bowl.

In a small cup, whisk lemon or lime juice, olive oil, and spices to make the dressing.

Finally, add the pita chips and if you like, add more sumacs and toss again. Transfer to small bowls or pans.

16. Mediterranean Couscous Salad

Ingredients

Couscous

   1 cup of water

   1 cup of couscous

   ½ teaspoon of salt

   2 tablespoons of virgin olive oil

Salad

   ½ cup of Roma tomato

   ½ cup of English cucumber

   ½ cup of red pepper

   ½ cup of garbanzo beans

   ½ cup of kalamata olives,

   2 tablespoons of feta cheese

   1 teaspoon of parsley

   ¼ cup of red onion

   1 teaspoon of mint

   1 teaspoon of basil

   ¼ teaspoon of oregano

Lemon Dressing

   1 teaspoon of lemon zest

   2 tablespoons of lemon juice

   1 tablespoon of red wine vinegar

   ¼ teaspoon of salt

   ¼ teaspoon of black pepper

3 tablespoons of olive oil

Directions

In a medium casserole dish, put water, salt, and olive oil to a boil. Add the couscous and mix fast. Switch the heat off and cover.

Let your couscous stand tender and fluff with a fork for 5 minutes and let it cool.

Salad

In a medium bowl, mix couscous, tomatoes, cucumber, beans, garbanzo, red onion, olives, cheese, Persil, mince, basil, and oregano.

Citrus Dressing

Whisk together the lemon rind, lemon juice, vinegar, salt, and pepper in a small cup. Drizzle slowly in olive oil and whisk until thickened.

Pour over the couscous salad, blend. Mix well.

In a medium casserole, put water, salt, and olive oil to a boil. Add the couscous and mix fast. Switch the heat off and cover.

Let your couscous stand tender and fluff with a fork for 5 minutes and let it cool.

17. Chicken Piccata

Ingredients

2 pcs of skinless chicken breasts,

A pinch of sea salt

Black pepper

6 tablespoons of butter unsalted

5 tablespoons of olive oil

1/3 cup of lemon juice

1/2 cup of chicken stock

All-purpose flour

1/4 cup of brined capers

1/3 cup of fresh parsley

Directions

Season chicken with salt and pepper.

Melt 2 tablespoons of butter in a wide saucepan over medium temperature with 3 tablespoons of olive oil. When oil and butter begin to sizzle, add 2 chicken pieces and cook 3 minutes. Cook on the other side for 3 minutes until the chicken is browned.

 Melt 2 more tablespoons of butter and add 2 more tablespoons of olive oil. When butter and oil start sizzling, add 2 chicken pieces and brown on both sides. Remove the bowl heat and add the chicken to it.

Add the citrus juice, pan, and stock capers. Return to the pot and carry the brown bits to a boil.

Put all the chicken back into the pot and cook for 5 minutes. Take the chicken to the plate from the dish. Stir in 2 tablespoons of butter and vigorously whisk. Sprinkle with chicken and parsley sauce.

18. Herb Crusted Turkey Tenderloin

Ingredients

  1 1⁄4 lbs. of skinless turkey tenderloins

  1 tablespoon of honey mustard

  1 tablespoon of lemon zest

  1 teaspoon of dried rosemary

  2 teaspoons of dried oregano

  Salt and pepper

Directions

Preheat the oven to 400 degrees Fahrenheit. Coat a shallow baker with a spray cooker.

Season turkey with pepper and salt

Place the sweet mustard over the turkey, then coat with rosemary zest and oregano.

Bake in the oven for 160 or about 35-40 minutes before the thermometer reads.

Let it rest approximately 10 minutes before slicing.

19. Oven-Roasted Turkey

Ingredients

1 tablespoon of paprika smoked

1 1/2 teaspoon of garlic powder

1 1/2 teaspoon of powdered onion

1 teaspoon of cayenne pepper

1 teaspoon of dried thyme

Kosher salt

Freshly ground black pepper

1 14-pound turkey

Olive oil

Fresh thyme

Directions

Mix smoked paprika in the bowl, onion powder, garlic powder, cayenne pepper, 1 tablespoon of salt, dried thyme, and 1 1/2 black pepper teaspoon. Within the turkey cavity, sprinkle some of the spice rubs.

Separate the skin with your fingers from breast meat, start from the top of the breast and slide left and right, then cook down.

Massage the meat with some of the mixture. Sprinkle it on the skin of the turkey. Place the turkey on a sheet of plastic wrap and cover—cool overnight or up to 24 hours to marry flavors.

Place a rack in the oven at the lowest level and heat to 325 degrees F. Remove the turkey from cold to room temperature. Hold the legs together and tuck the tips of the wing. Put the turkey in a roasting pan.

Drizzle olive oil outside the turkey and sprinkle with salt and pepper. Roast the turkey for 3 hours until the thermometer inserted into the thigh's thickest area is 165 degrees F.

Place the turkey on top of a platter and cover with foil loosely and let it remain for 30 minutes.

20. Tenderized Vinegar Chicken

180g chicken breast,

1/2 teaspoon of baking soda

Sauce

1 tablespoon of cornflour

1 1/2 tablespoon of soy sauce

1 tablespoon of Oyster Sauce

1 tablespoon of Cooking Wine

1/2 teaspoon of sesame oil

White pepper

3/4 cup of (185 ml) water

Stir Fry:

1 1/2 tablespoon of vegetable oil

2 pcs of garlic cloves

1/2 onion sliced

5 - 6 stems choy sum

1 medium carrot

1/2 cup of sliced mushrooms

Directions

Put the chicken inside a bowl and sprinkle it with baking soda. Use your fingers to mix and store for 20 minutes for no more than 30 minutes (can get too tender). Rinse well, remove excess water with paper towels.

Ingredients

Sauce: Cornflour and soy sauce in a tub. Mix

Apply the remaining sauce ingredients and blend.

Chop choy sum: Then split into 7cm pieces (3")—separate stems of the trees.

Break the carrot into 3-cm bits (1.3") then slice the bits thinly.

Stir Fry:

Heat olive oil over high heat. Add garlic, stir rapidly, add onion, cook 1 minute and change continuously until onion begins to wipe.

Add the chicken and cook till the surface turns pink to white for 1 minute.

Add choy sum, carrot, and champagne. Stir in the saucepan for 1 minute.

Add choy sum leaves, sparkling bean, and sauce. Stir-fry for 1 to 2 minutes until the sauce is thick to a thick syrup. Vegetables should be tender/crisp.

Serve immediately with rice; try cauliflower rice for low carb, low cal alternative!

21. Herb Roasted Chicken Breast

Ingredients

3 tablespoons of butter

2 cloves garlic

1 teaspoon of dried basil

1 teaspoon of dried thyme

1 teaspoon of dried rosemary

1/2 teaspoon of salt

Freshly cracked black pepper

2 split chicken breasts

Directions

Preheat oven to 275F. Remove the chicken from the refrigerator and let the butter mix warm slightly for 5 minutes or so.

Stir butter, sliced garlic, basil, thyme, rosemary, salt, and pepper in a small cup. Rosemary pieces can be very large, so chop the dried parts with your hands until they are added to the mix.

Place the chicken on a cutting board and pat with a clean towel on both sides. Rub the chicken butter herb mixture on both sides. The drying of the meat helps to stick the butter herb. If the meat is too cold, it develops condensation when the butter blend is rubbed over the surface, and the butter does not stick.

In a casserole dish that is deep enough to hold the entire chicken, put the seasoned chicken bits. Cover closely with foil or, if one exists, with the dish's lid. Bake the chicken for 90 minutes in the preheated oven and grill halfway through once.

Remove the foil after 90 minutes, rub and raise the oven's temperature to 425F again. Bake the chicken without a foil at 425 F for around 20 minutes or until the skin is deep brown and crispy. Remove the chicken from the oven and allow 5-10 minutes to rest.

Pull the meat from the bone or slice the breasts. Conserve the juices from the casserole dish and drizzle it on the meat.

22. Sole With Herbed Butter

Ingredients

Dill sprigs

1/2 cup of butter

2 tablespoons of chives

1 tablespoon of dill

1 tablespoon of thyme

Olive oil

1 tablespoon of lemon juice

4- to 5-ounce sole fillets

Lemon wedges

Directions

In a small cup, mix the butter, chopped herbs, and fresh lemon juice—season with salt and pepper to taste.

Preheat grill. On the rimmed baking sheet, put the fish fillets, brush them with olive oil, and sprinkle salt and pepper. Broil in the center about 3 minutes. Spoon butter mixture over fish. Broil just about 1 minute longer before butter melts. Move fish to plates, spoon melted butter over fillets from a tray. Add dill sprigs and wedges of lemon and serve.

23. Lemon Rosemary Salmon

Ingredients

  1 thinly sliced lemon,

  4 sprigs rosemary

  2 salmon fillets

Salt to taste

  1 tablespoon of olive oil

Directions

Preheat the oven to 200 degrees Celsius

Arrange half of the lemon slices in one layer of a baking dish, add 2 rosemary layer sprigs and cover with salmon fillets. Sprinkle with salt, cover with the rest of the citrus fruit, layer with remaining sprigs. Sprinkle olive oil.

Bake inside a preheated oven for 20 minutes until the fish flakes easily with a fork.

24. Tuna Melt Zucchini Boats

Ingredients

   1 large zucchini

   Kosher salt

Pepper,

   ½ red onion

   1 5oz can of tuna

   1 celery stalk

   ¼ cup of Greek yogurt

   2 tablespoon of dill

   1 tablespoon of lemon juice

   1 jalapeno

   1 teaspoon of Dijon mustard

   ¼ cup of cheddar cheese

Optional toppings

   Red chili peppers

   Corn

   Chopped tomatoes

   Green onions

Directions

Preheat your oven to 350F and add a baking parchment paper.

Break the zucchini half longitudinally, scoop out the inside and save for further use.

In the prepared baking tray, put the zucchini and spray with the cooking oil. Season to taste with salt and pepper, then place into an oven's middle rack, and cook for 12-15 minutes until tender.

Add salmon, celery, red onion, yogurt, dill, mustard, citrus juice, and jalapeño in a mixing bowl. Mix, then taste and season as required with salt and pepper.

Then brush the courgettes with the tuna mixture with the cheddar.

Bake for about 10 minutes until cheese is melted.

25. Baked Cod

Ingredients

   3 dashes cayenne pepper

   1/4 teaspoon of salt

   1 tablespoon of lemon juice

   1 1/2 tablespoon of olive oil

   1 tablespoon of parsley

   1 lb. cod fillets

Directions

Preheat to 400F in the oven.

Arrange the cod fillets then drizzle the olive oil and the salt lemon juice, and cayenne pepper into the fish.

Bake the cod for 10-12 minutes in the oven, depending on the cod's thickness. Garnish with parsley and serve as soon as possible.

26. Mushroom Florentine Pasta

Ingredients

    8 ounces linguine pasta,

    3 tablespoons of all-purpose flour

    8 ounces chicken broth

    8 ounces whole milk

    1/2 teaspoon of salt

    1/2 teaspoon of black pepper

    1.5 ounces (3 tablespoons of) olive oil

    8 ounces (weight) mushrooms

    2 garlic cloves

    3 ounces (weight) Gruyere cheese shredded

    2 cups of baby spinach leaves

Directions

Start cooking pasta as instructed in the box.

Whisk chicken broth, milk, salt, and pepper together. Set aside.

During pasta cooking, heat olive oil over medium-high heat in a large skillet. Add sliced mushrooms when oil starts to ripple, sauté for 6 minutes. Add thin garlic and sprinkle for another 2 minutes until garlic is brown.

Whisk in mushrooms and garlic; add chicken broth, milk, pepper, salt mixture, simmer, and cook, occasionally stirring until thickened, approximately 3-4 minutes.

Stir until cheese has melted; add shredded cheese.

Add drained pasta to the saucepan and toss to coat.

27. Sweet Potato Balls

Ingredients

   1 lb. of sweet potatoes

   ¾ to 1 cup of white rice flour

   ¼ cup of sugar

   1 teaspoon of baking powder

   ½ cup of rice flour

   Vegetable oil

Directions

Peel and cube sweet potatoes. Set in a steamer and steam until soft for 10 minutes. Put the potato mash in a large dish.

In sweet potatoes, add rice and flour, seed sugar, and baking powder. Mix to form smooth dough. Apply a white meal of rice while the dough is still very tender. The dough needs to be smooth.

Take the dough out of the bowl to form a 1-inch ball between your hands. Repeat until all the dough is used.

Please add 1 inch of vegetable oil to the medium pot over medium-low heat. Drop a couple of sweet potato balls into the hot oil gently. Fry until golden brown for 3 to 4 minutes. When fried, sweet potato balls will float. Remove the tongs on a wire strainer and drain them. Repeat until all sweet balls of potato are fried.

Serve immediately.

28. Shepherd's Pie

Filling

Ingredients

　1 medium onion

　2 cloves of garlic

　1 1/2 cup of uncooked brown lentils

　4 cups of vegetable stock

　2 teaspoons of thyme

　1 10-ounce bag of frozen mixed veggies

Potatoes Mashed

　3 pounds of gold potatoes

　3-4 tablespoons of vegan butter

Pepper and salt

Directions

Cut the big potatoes in half, place them in a big pot, and fill with water. Cover and cook for 20-30 minutes.

When the water is heated, drain off the remaining water from the pot. Use a big fork to smoothly mash. Add the desired quantity of vegan butter (3-4 slices of salt and pepper as the initial recipe is prepared/modified if batch size changes). Cover and set loosely aside.

Plate a baking dish for two quarters of a time.

Sprinkle and cook the onions and the garlic into a large casserole of olive oil until slightly brownish and caramelized, around 5 minutes.

Apply a pinch of salt and pepper. Stir in the stock and thyme. Take a medium simmer, take a low boil. Reduce to cool. Continue to cook until the lens is tender (35-40 minutes).

During the last 10 minutes of cooking, mix, and combine the frozen vegetables.

OPTIONAL: Add mash potatoes to thicken the mixture. Scoop 1/2 blend and whisk into 2 cups.

Return to the pot and thicken the whisk.

Adjust seasoning and taste accordingly. Take the prepared oven-safe baking dish and cover it with pumpkin carefully. Smooth with a spoon or fork and apply some sea salt to the pepper.

Place on a baking sheet and bake for 10-15 minutes or untilslightly browned mashers.

Let it cool briefly before serving. The longer it lies, the more it becomes heavier. Cool before covering, then store in the refrigerator for a few days.

29. Double Choc Vanilla Brownies

Ingredients

   200g of cooking chocolate

   200g of unsalted butter

   3 large eggs,

   3 teaspoons Vanilla Bean Paste

   1 cup of (150g) plain flour

   1/4 cup of (30g) cocoa powder

   1 cup of (220g) caster sugar

   250g white chocolate

Directions

Preheat the oven up to 170°C (fan-forced). Line the bottom and sides of a 20cm square pastry bowl with baking paper.

In a microwave, put dark chocolate and butterfor about 30 seconds, stirring between them until the chocolate has melted. Two-three minutes. In chocolate mixture and whisk, add eggs, sugar, and vanilla bean paste.

Combine flour and cocoa in a separate dish. Gradually blend the chocolate mixture with a whisk. Remove the pieces of white chocolate and pour the batter into the prepared pot. Bake until the crumbs adhere to a skewer inserted in the middle of the brownies for 40 minutes. Remove from the oven and cool in a saucepan before chopping.

To freeze, simply allow brownies to cool completely in the clinging wrap and freeze for up to 3 months.

30. Grilled Peaches

Ingredients

4 halved and pitted ripe peaches

1 tablespoon of vegetable oil

Vanilla ice cream

Honey

Flaky sea salt

Directions

Heat grill to medium-high

Brush the peaches and grill gently for 4 to 5 minutes.

Flip your skin and grill nearly 4 to 6 more minutes before you break down.

Serve with ice cream, salt, and honey from a sprinkler of sweet seafood.

CHAPTER 8:
FREQUENTLY ASKED QUESTIONS

A recent review indicated that this popular beverage does not increase the longer-lasting risk of high blood pressure or heart disease, although the increase in blood pressure was short-term (1-3 hours)

• Do I need a DASH diet practice?

It is recommended that you do 30 minutes of moderate activity for most days, and it is important to choose something that you like – in this way, you will more likely keep it up.

DASH diet is even more effective at decreasing blood pressure if combined with physical activity. Examples of moderate exercise include, rustic walking (15 minutes per mile or 9 minutes per kilometer), running (10 minutes per mile or 6 minutes per km), cycling (6 minutes/mile or 4 minutes/km) (60 minutes)

• Can I drink alcohol while on a DASH diet?

Too much alcohol can increase your blood pressure; in fact, it's associated with an increased risk of high blood pressure and heart disease to regularly drink more than three drinks a day. On the DASH diet, it is 2 or less for men, and 1 or fewer for women; you are required to drink alcohol sparingly.

• Is the DASH diabetes diet safe?

In contrast to often difficult to maintain faded diets, the DASH diet—which has long been promoted for its advantages in lowering high blood pressure—is also a top choice for diabetes care and is easy to begin. Let's look at what distinguishes it.

DASH stands for Dietary Approaches Stop Hypertension. Its main objective is to reduce blood pressure. Diabetes and high blood pressure tend to go hand in hand: over half of all adults with diabetes are diagnosed with hypertension. DASH diet may improve insulin resistance, high blood pressure and hyperlipidemia (an abnormally high fat concentration in the blood), and obesity.

It works well on prediabetes and type 1 and types 2 diabetes because of diet on weight, insulin sensitivity, and glycemic control. Research on the diabetes spectrum shows that the diet can reduce the future risk of type 2 diabetes by 20 percent.

• Is DASH the same diet as Keto?

The Whole30, Dukan, and Keto diets are more restrictive on foods than DASH and the Mediterranean diets. This can make it harder for them to follow in the long run.

What is the DASH Diet Plan?

The DASH diet is essential for nutritional methods to avoid high blood pressure. People are also put on this diet at the start of hypertension to help control blood pressure.

The plan is focused on 2,000 calories a day but can be changed to suit any dietary requirements. The American Heart Association strongly recommends this diet to maintain good health in many ways other than hypertension. Naturally, the essential elements to support hypertension include foods that are high in potassium, calcium-containing foods, and magnesium as well.

First of all, the DASH strategy puts a great deal of emphasis on grains. With 7-8 servings a day, it is smart to have whole wheat loaves of bread, wheat pasta, and whole-grain cereals. All your grains have much more nutritional qualities than other grains that hold more refined sugar.

The DASH diet also promotes fruits and vegetables. This category allows you to eat 4 to 5 portions a day. The guide tells you some excellent ways to include your portions of fruits and vegetables every day.

Next to this strategy are non-fat or low-fat dairy products. You'll need to select skim milk, or 1% at most, cheese and yogurt that is low-fat or fat. You have lean meat options after milk. You get small portion sizes, not more than 2 parts. Healthy options include skinless chicken, fatty frankfurters, and other lean foods.

When you get to the section where the plan addresses nuts and seeds, they cannot exceed five small portions a week. This included legumes as well.

As you need to adjust the plan to your daily calories, it will teach you how. The book also will teach you about healthy ways to feed. When on a diet plan, eating out is a real challenge, but the DASH Diet book will greatly tell you how.

The plan has a portion of the book that talks about workouts and alcoholic drinks and ways to help you get away from smoking. Such medical conditions for which this approach seems helpful are insulin resistance, cholesterol, and inflammation. If you have trouble with any of these medical problems other than hypertension, take this meal plan seriously.

DASH is a nutritional strategy for stopping high blood pressure. The DASH diet has been scientifically shown to reduce blood pressure in people within 2 weeks of the diet. It is popular to control blood pressure and prevent cardiovascular diseases, stroke, diabetes, and some types of cancer.

The Target

The NHLBI conducted a series of studies and research on certain dietary patterns or diets. The use of less fat, cholesterol, sodium, and more whole grains, fruits, vegetables, and low-fat dairy products helped reduce blood pressure.

The Eating Plan should be adopted as a better approach to managing the condition and the overall balanced body rather than as a strict weight loss plan.

Below are the tips proposed by the DASH diet

Eat a heavy breakfast, heavier than normal, but choose a safer choice than a refined and sweetened one, for example, whole grain cereals. You don't want to do that during the day.

Double the servings of fruits and vegetables

Reduce the usual fat intake by half or choose the low fat or non-fat types.

Search for sweets, fruit snacks, or raw edible vegetables.

Remove sodium from your diet slowly.

Choose white over red portions when you want to eat meat.

Never try to make any drastic changes; do so in paces to prevent dietary crashes that are very unhealthy.

Although it was originally conceived and aimed to control and lower blood pressure rather than for purposes of losing weight, with a few adjustments, it can easily be tailored to control weight as well.

Who should follow the DASH food plan?

A DASH food plan will potentially be part of every balanced food plan. It lowers blood pressure and provides more health benefits, including decreased LDL cholesterol and inflammation.

How does the food plan DASH work?

The diet consists of some nutrient-rich foods, including potassium, calcium, and magnesium, which minimize blood pressure. The diet is high in fiber that lowers blood pressure and removes the extra kilograms to relieve blood pressure.

What do you eat on a DASH food plan?

The grains are bundled with nutrients including protein, vitamins and trace minerals, fiber, and antioxidants, such as whole wheat, brown rice, oats, barley, quinoa. However, in refined grains, most nutrients are lacking and should be avoided.

Please include fat or fat-free milk, yogurt, Greek yogurt, breadcrumbs, and not all fat choices in your diet. Milk and dairy products without lactose are a choice for people who are intolerant to lactose.

Nuts such as almonds, walnuts, pistachios, etc., beans, dals, and seeds such as seeds of sunflower, melon, etc., are part of a balanced diet of DASH for food. They contain high fiber, omega-3 fatty acids, vitamins, and minerals, such as zinc and magnesium. While nuts contain healthy fats, they should be eaten in small amounts.

Stop salt or honey-roasted nuts due to their high sodium and sugar content.

Instead of high-saturated fat meats, lean meat, eggs, poultry, and fish are mild. Processed meats such as bacon, ham, sausages, salamis, etc., contain considerable sodium, restricting the intake. The eating of red meat is tolerated from time to time.

Of course, potassium is rich in fruits and vegetables, which help lower blood pressure very effectively. Adjust it gradually if you don't like fruit and vegetables. In addition to what youalready have, add extra fruit or vegetable to the supply in the day. I prefer the whole fruit to juices.

Unsweetened dried fruits such as raisins, cannibals, dried figs, etc., are fine travel choices. Ensure that each meal has a vegetable.

The diet should have low saturated fats and total fats. High saturated fat intakes increase the risk of cardiovascular disease and high blood pressure. Fats are important for absorption and help to produce fat-soluble vitamins in the body's immune system. Any meal can prevent oils such as olive oil, rice bran oil, motor oil, and trans fats widely used in processed and fried food.

Reducing alcohol intake can help lower blood pressure. Keep alcohol intake under control.

Aerobic exercise and DASH diet work to lower blood pressure more efficiently.

Read food labels to choose products that are less sodium.

Stress will raise blood pressure even if you are healthy with your diet. Stress control techniques such as meditation, yoga, etc., will also help to control blood pressure.

The pressure of the blood increases because of insufficient sleep. Sound sleep helps control blood pressure for seven to eight hours.

Cutting them will help lower blood pressure if you are someone who smokes.

Take the medication you prescribe.

Limit salt intake to 1 tea cubicle per day.

It's an attempt to change your lifestyle. It is a long-term commitment to good health. Smaller adjustments will deliver faster results than dramatic changes and lose the effort on the way. Before joining the DASH diet, visit a nutritionist.

DASH's high blood pressure diet is the most prescribed diet for hypertension patients for years. Many scientists and organizations, especially the National Institutes of Health, have studied it extensively. Instead of merely lowering sodium, the DASH HP diet continues, offering a balanced nutritious way to eat little calories and at the same time, plenty vitamins, minerals, and fibers.

However, it can be difficult to make the requisite adjustments to adopt the DASH diet without certain limitations after a lifetime. Here are five tips that will motivate you to implement this strategy in your everyday life.

Just because you limit your salt consumption, it doesn't mean your food is bland and tasteless. Try adding a range of herbs and spices to your food to improve the taste without adding sodium. Herbs and spices are very low in calories and high in taste. Create your mixtures of herbs and spices for rubbing, adding soups, and preparing your favorite recipes.

Eat a balanced snack

When you're away from your kitchen, it can be very difficult to eat well. When you're at work, the temptation to reach the nearby distributor can be high if you start to be hungry. Instead, carrya tiny bag of unsalted nuts or a nutritious snack like carrot or celery sticks.

Replace your meat

Legumes are a big replacement for high-pressure DASH beef. They are savory but without all the added fat that accompanies many meat cuts. They also provide a lot of protein and fiber that keeps you full after you eat them.

Enjoy desserts

Face it - every single one of us has one or two sweet teeth, and desserts are always the first items to go on a diet. The DASH

High Blood Pressure Diet suggests 4-5 portions of fruit a day to create your dessert. Fresh strawberries with some fat cream create a great, satisfying, and fatty dessert.

Fit the plants in

Gardens are one of the pillars of your new way of eating, so you have to find ways to adapt them to any meal. Taste your sandwich with low sodium tomato juice, add lettuce, onions, and tomato, and have a wonderful vegetable with dinner. The trick is to try new things regularly, so you don't get bored.

You will begin to experience a decrease in your hypertension in a few weeks if you adopt the DASH high blood pressure diet. As with every new food plan, the trick to following it is finding ways to put it into your particular timetable and match your personal needs.

There are also things that you can do naturally to relieve blood pressure. If you begin to exhibit elevated blood pressure signs, start taking an aggressive approach immediately.

CONCLUSION

Today, the lifestyles we live are very different from those of our ancestors. With the invasion of technology, we are becoming increasingly busy, and our lives are full of stress and tension, and some rely on the way we eat and what we eat.

In reality, the word DASH means diet approaches to avoid high blood pressure. It is promoted by the National Institute of Health, a government agency in the United States. DASH itself explains that the DASH diet is specifically used to control high blood pressure. Currently, about 50 million people in the U.S. and around 1 billion worldwide are affected by hypertension.

The link between cardiovascular and blood pressure remains constant. There is a higher risk that heart attack events, heart failure, heart stroke, and other kidney diseases may occur.

Diet and exercise will only improve our muscle strength, but the probability of such an occurrence cannot be minimized. If anyone has hypertension, their body will not respond much to their health, so we must care for muscle and intellectual organs.

One of the DASH diet's main elements is restricting sodium and nuts, whole grains, fish, meat, fruit, and vegetables. DASH Diet also advocates the reduction of red meat, sweets, and sugar intake. A diet rich in potassium, magnesium, calcium, protein, and fiber is DASH.

The diet helps to minimize the systolic blood pressure and diastolic pressure in patients by having a daily intake of calories from 1699 to 3100. Since DASH's diet has a high antioxidant content, it can help prevent chronic health issues such as cancer, cardiac disorders, and stroke.

Initially, this diet was developed in 1992 to find the right diet to tackle increased morbid hypertension among Americans.

Today, after years of careful tests performed by various public health agencies, the United States government promoted the DASH diet to prevent lifestyle diseases in people with high blood pressure and as a safe diet model to any American.

The diet for DASH supports more fruits, vegetables, whole grains, and low-fat dairy products. The diet also includes margarine, fish, poultry, nuts, and beans as various protein sources and recommends salt, sugar, and fats, in general, to be reduced.

The maximum amount of salt per day was 3,200 mg from all sources. Just three teaspoons were limited to sugar. Alcohol intake is limited to no more than two drinks, and coffee and cola are limited to a total of three drinks a day.

Although not completely vegetarian, studies of people using the DASH model will significantly reduce blood pressure by 6 mm Hg in systolic and 3 mm Hg in diastolic in ordinary people. For hypertensive citizens, 11 mm Hg and 6 mm Hg respectively are decreased.

This is done to avoid further complications, such as cardiac insufficiency, kidney failure, coronary heart disease, and blood vessel hardening. It was universal for men and women between 48 and 83 years of age.

This diet is easy to follow but be cautious of so-called balanced foods that conceal large quantities of salt, white sugar, and fats. See packaging for sodium tubes, maize syrups, and saturated fats. DASH diet retains a healthier body weight than conform to fads that promise drastic weight loss.

The United States National Heart, Lung, and Blood Institute has long advocated a dash diet to manage high blood pressure. The dash diet or a nutritional strategy to avoid high blood pressure is a diet that reduces sodium intake.

The diet supports whole food, fruit and vegetables, fish and poultry, and nuts. Red meat and sweets intake is a total taboo if you closely observe the DASH diet. The diet is also rich in magnesium, calcium, carbohydrate, magnesium, and potassium, essential for good health. The dash diet focuses primarily on controlling blood pressure below 120/80 mmHg.

While the DASH diet is not technically vegetarian, it promotes fruit, nuts, and beans to consume rather than meats. Processed foods and junk foods in this diet are completely not recommended. There are safe substitute snacks to fill this space by satisfying this sweet tooth.

The N.I.H. published a guidebook titled, "Your Guide to Lowering Your Blood Pressure with Dash," which gives details of the diet and also a list of how to get the required food to start with. It also offers guidelines on the quantities and substitute foods to be eaten in the diet.

It was shown that the diet would decrease systolic blood pressure by 6 mm Hg. Diagnostic blood pressure of 3 mm Hg also has been shown to minimize normal blood pressure in diets. Hypertension has also been known to decrease with diet from 11 to 6.

The use of the diet in time is often thought to reduce stroke and heart disease risk. The proper use of the DASH diet lowers blood pressure and other elevated blood pressure problems and provides catering advantages beyond what anyone ever expected. In all of this, the diet also requires you to eat between 1699 and 3100 dietary calories a day!

This diet is high in fiber, so some people may have diarrhea and bloom. However, to address this, the amount of fruit, vegetable, and whole-grain consumed can be increased.

It is important to be aware because too many fibers can also cause constipation if you don't drink enough water, so ensure you drink a lot.

CPSIA information can be obtained
at www.ICGtesting.com
Printed in the USA
LVHW030914210121
676963LV00005B/300

9 781914 163340